Caring for You
  ∽ *Caring for Me*

Caring for You ~ Caring for Me

Education and Support for Caregivers

Participant's Manual

Developed by

David H. Haigler, Ed.D.
Kathryn B. Mims, Ph.D.
Jack A. Nottingham, Ph.D.

Rosalynn Carter Institute
Georgia Southwestern State University

Copyright 1998 Rosalynn Carter Institute
Georgia Southwestern State University
Americus, GA 31709
All rights reserved

ISBN 0-8203-2043-9

02 01 00 99 98   5 4 3 2 1

Distributed by:
The University of Georgia Press
330 Research Drive, Athens, GA 30602-4901
Telephone: 1-800-266-5842
FAX: 706-369-6131
E-mail: books@ugapress.uga.edu

Also available from the University of Georgia Press:

Caring for You, Caring for Me: Education and Support for Caregivers. Leader's Guide, developed by David H. Haigler, Kathryn B. Mims, Jack A. Nottingham. ISBN: 0-8203-2042-0 (pa.)

Caring and Competent Caregivers by Robert M. Moroney, Paul R. Dokecki, John J. Gates, Kelly Noser Haynes, J. R. Newbrough, Jack A. Nottingham; with contributions from Pam Davis, David H. Haigler, Anne G. McWilliams, and David L. Smith. Preface by Rosalynn Carter. Foreword by Julius B. Richmond, M.D. ISBN 0-8203-1951-1 (cl.), 0-8203-1952-X (pa.)

Cover: Artist Julia LaPine, represented by Carolyn Potts and Associates, Chicago, Illinois

Contents

Introduction   1

Modules

Module 1: *What It Means to Be a Caregiver*   3
Module 2: *Taking Care of Yourself*   13
Module 3: *Building Cooperative Relationships*   27
Module 4: *Preventing and Solving Problems*   35
Module 5: *Accessing and Developing Resources*   41

Appendices

A. The Rosalynn Carter Institute   49
B. Suggested Readings for Formal and Informal Caregivers   51
C. National Sources of Help for Caregivers   83

The Authors   101

Introduction

~

Welcome to *Caring for You, Caring for Me: Education and Support for Caregivers*. This manual was designed to give you information and assistance as you participate in the education and support program. It contains course materials, class exercises, and reference materials.

The *Caring for You, Caring for Me* program was developed by the Rosalynn Carter Institute of Georgia Southwestern State University in Americus, Georgia. A description of the Institute may be found in Appendix A. The broad objectives of the *Caring for You, Caring for Me* program are for caregivers to have the opportunity to:

- gain information on various topics related to caregiving
- learn ways of coping with the stresses and strains of being a caregiver
- learn what resources are available locally, regionally, and nationally
- discover ways of working together to reduce some of the frustrations and barriers of the caregiving role
- share common concerns
- recognize that others share similar feelings and concerns

The program is divided into five topics, or modules:

- What It Means to Be a Caregiver
- Taking Care of Yourself
- Building Cooperative Relationships
- Preventing and Solving Problems
- Accessing and Developing Resources

The Participant's Manual is organized into five sections—one for each module. Each section contains the informational guides which support the presentation by the program leader(s) and pages to be completed in class exercises. The manual also contains a suggested reading list for caregivers (Appendix B) and a list of national sources of help for caregivers (Appendix C).

In order to get the most from this program, it is recommended that you follow instructions of the program leader(s) as to how to use this manual. You are especially encouraged to wait for instructions from the leader before completing any of the forms or exercises in the manual.

MODULE 1
What It Means to Be a Caregiver

Purposes of Session

The purposes of this session are:

- to introduce participants to the *Caring for You, Caring for Me* program.
- to define "caregiving" and "caregiver."
- to help participants understand the importance of caregivers, the need for care, the nature of the caring relationship, and the rewards and difficulties faced by caregivers.
- to encourage sharing of individual caregiving situations among participants in order to gain understanding of and support for each other.

INFORMATION SHEET

NAME:

MAILING ADDRESS:

DAYTIME TELEPHONE:
_____

1. What is your occupation or major pastime?

2. Whom do you care for? Why do they need care?

3. How did you become a caregiver?

Types of Caregivers

1. **Formal (professional) caregivers** provide health care or social service to others as a part of their profession using skills, knowledge and insight gained through formal training; they are usually paid for their service. Examples: a nurse in a home health care agency; a social worker in a mental health program; a nurse's aide in a nursing home.

2. **Informal (lay or family) caregivers** provide care and assistance to others, usually as part of an ongoing relationship as an expression of concern and love . . . for a relative, friend or neighbor, without financial or material gain.

3. **Volunteer caregivers** may be considered as formal or informal depending upon the formal training received and specific job as a volunteer.
    a. Example (formal): a nurse who works for a hospice (as a nurse) with no pay.
    b. Example (informal): a congregational volunteer who visits elderly persons and "shut-ins" as part of an ongoing congregational-supported program.

4. **Dual caregivers** provide care for family members or relatives in addition to their professional roles and responsibilities.

Health Situations Creating the Need for Care

Physical illnesses or disabilities

Mental illnesses

Developmental disabilities

Substance abuse

Difficulties of the frail elderly

National Trends Affecting Caregiving

People are Living Longer

* Life expectancy (at birth) has increased from 47 years in 1900 to 68 in 1950 to 76 years in 1995.

* In 1992, there were 32.3 million persons who were 65 years old or older living in the United States (12.7% of the total population). This number has increased 10 times (from 3.1 million) and the percentage has more than tripled (from 4.1%) since 1900.

* By the year 2030 the number of persons 65 years old and older is expected to reach 70 million, or 20% of the total population.

* The fastest growing age group is made up of persons over 85 years old.

* The dramatic increase in some diseases is at least partially due to longer life. (Examples include prostate cancer in men over 70 and Alzheimer's disease).

Advances in Medical Technology

* More people at all ages whose conditions would have caused death are now able to live with the availability of new technologies and treatments.

* Medical technology has improved survival rates but increased the need for care over long periods of time.

Increased Need for Care

* It is estimated that over 11 million children and adults are either physically or mentally disabled and need care or support services.

* The number of persons needing care is expected to triple by 2025.

continued

Shift in Where Care is Provided

* The main location of care has moved out of hospitals and institutions and into homes and communities.

* Persons are being discharged from hospitals "quicker and sicker."

* Efforts to decrease costs of medical care have resulted in an increased reliance on unpaid (informal) caregivers to provide care for persons with illnesses and disabilities.

* 70 to 90% of care is provided by informal caregivers (mostly family members and other relatives).

Changes in Families

* Women continue to provide most of the care at home—approximately 80% of informal caregivers are women.

* More than half of all married women are employed outside the home, and the number continues to increase.

* There has been an increase in single-parent families, resulting from a combination of the rising number of single women bearing children and the growing divorce rate.

* Families tend to be more geographically mobile, resulting in more distance between family members.

* Families have become more "verticalized"—an increasing number of living generations, with a decreasing number of persons within each generation.

What Is Known About Caregiving and Caregivers

~

According to research by numerous experts and scholars, all caregivers are at risk of certain types of strain and distress because of the following factors:

* Time consumed in personal care.

* Financial costs associated with disability or illness.

* Stigma associated with certain illnesses or difficulties.

* Conflicting roles and values.

* Difficulties in physical management such as lifting and assisting with movement.

* Interruption of sleep.

* Social isolation and limitation of recreational activities.

* Management of behavior problems.

* Limited prospects for the future.

Elements of Caring*

~

Knowledge

Understanding the care receiver's needs, powers, and limitations.

Patience

Letting the care receiver grow in his or her own time.

Honesty

Being genuine; seeing the care receiver as he or she really is,
and not how you would like them to be.

Trust

Allowing the care receiver freedom to make choices (and mistakes) and
not "overprotecting";
Trusting your capacity to care.

Humility

Always ready and willing to learn more about the care receiver.

Hope

Appreciation of the present as alive with possibilities for the future.

Courage

Taking risks; moving into the future with confidence and the insight gained from
past and present experiences.

---

*From Mayerhoff, M. (1971). *On Caring*. Scranton, PA: HarperCollins.

Principles That Guide *Caring for You, Caring for Me*

1. **Genuine concern for the person receiving care.**

    * A basic assumption for both formal or informal caregivers.

    * A must for adequate quality of care.

2. **Need to take care of self—as a caregiver.**

    * Avoid becoming a casualty, also in need of care.

    * Results in better and longer care for care receiver.

3. **Commonality among caregivers.**

    * Caregivers for persons with various kinds of difficulties have common needs and concerns.

    * Caregivers will benefit by coming together to address their common concerns.

4. **Mutuality between formal and informal caregivers.**

    * Formal and informal caregivers have mutual concerns and strengths that complement each other.

    * The care receivers will ultimately receive better care if formal and informal caregivers work together as a caregiving team.

MODULE 2
Taking Care of Yourself

Purposes of Session

The purposes of this session are:

* to help participants learn how to assess their "self-care" skills.
* to identify outcomes of NOT taking care of oneself.
* to identify and examine negative emotions.
* to identify effective coping skills.
* to examine personal support systems.
* to recognize the role and importance of humor and laughter.

Do You Take Care of Yourself? Assessment for Caregivers*

Rate each item below from 1 (almost always) to 5 (never), according to how much of the time each statement applies to you.

1 = Almost Always   3 = Occasionally
2 = Frequently   4 = Rarely
5 = Never

	RATING
1. I exercise on a regular basis.	1 2 3 4 5
2. I make and keep preventive and necessary medical and dental appointments.	1 2 3 4 5
3. I have a job or regular volunteer activity that is gratifying.	1 2 3 4 5
4. I do not use tobacco products.	1 2 3 4 5
5. I do not use alcohol or drugs.	1 2 3 4 5
6. I get an adequate amount of sleep each day.	1 2 3 4 5
7. I have a hobby or recreational activity I enjoy and spend time doing.	1 2 3 4 5
8. I eat at least two to three balanced meals a day.	1 2 3 4 5
9. I have at least one person in whom I can confide (tell all my problems, discuss my successes).	1 2 3 4 5
10. I take time to do things that are important to me (e.g., go to church, spend time alone, garden, read)	1 2 3 4 5
11. I do not have problems with sleeplessness or anxiety.	1 2 3 4 5
12. I have personal goals and am taking steps to achieve them.	1 2 3 4 5
Total Score	

Add the numbers you placed at end of each item.

Interpretation:
    A total score of 12 to 24—You are doing an excellent job of taking care of yourself.
    A total score of 25 to 36—You have some room for improvement.
    A total score of 37 to 48—You are doing a poor job of taking care of yourself and are at moderately high risk for personal health problems.
    A total score of 48 to 60—You are at extremely high risk.

---

*Adapted from "Checklist For Caregivers: Do You Take Care of Yourself" (Bass, 1990, p. 35)
Bass, D. S. (1990). *Caring families: Supports and interventions*. Silver Spring, MD: National Association of Social Workers.

Some Causes & Symptoms of Caregiver Burnout

CAUSES

Conflicting demands from care receivers and others in the environment

The apparent helplessness of the care receiver's condition

Ambiguity of role(s)

Work load

Conflicting policies and procedures

⬇

which can lead to feelings of

LACK OF MASTERY
LACK OF AUTONOMY
FAILURE TO ACHIEVE GOALS

⬇

SYMPTOMS

Depression	Sleep
Withdrawal	Abuse from or of care receiver(s)
Feelings of helplessness or hopelessness	Neglect of care receiver(s)
Personal health problems	Negative emotions
Lowered self-esteem	Physical fatigue

Ways to Prevent Caregiver Burnout

1. Recognize and cope with your negative emotions.
2. Develop a battery of coping skills.
3. Don't go it alone. Let others help you.
4. Learn to laugh!

Common "Hooks"

~

"Hooks" are the things others do and/or say in efforts to manipulate us. In other words, "hooks" are what others use to get certain reactions from us, to get us off center and to use us. Some of the most common "hooks," and examples of each, include:

1. **Guilt/shame**
("If you really cared, you'd . . .")

2. **Blaming**
("You told me to . . . I did and look what happened." "It's all your fault.")

3. **Scapegoat**
("You expect too much of me.")

4. **Lack of empathy**
("You just don't know what I'm going through.")

5. **Advice seeking**
("I'm at my wit's end. What should I do?")

6. **Getting you to take sides**
("How could she have done this to me? She never has loved me, has she?")

Coping with "Negative" Emotions

A. Circle the one "negative" emotion that you experience most often or with which you have the greatest difficulty coping. If the negative emotion you experience most often is not listed, you may add it in the space provided.

Anger	Shame	Jealousy	Guilt
Depression	Frustration	Helplessness	_____
Inadequacy	Resentment	Sadness	
Failure	Fear	Loneliness	

B. Next answer the following questions about the emotion you circled.

1. When or under what circumstances do you tend to feel _____? (Be specific)

2. Who else is usually involved when you feel this way?

3. When was the last time you felt _____? Briefly describe exactly what happened.

4. What could you do to change the circumstances or situations in which you tend to feel _____? That is, what can you do to keep from feeling this way? (Be specific)

Coping Skills for Caregivers: A Summary

Stress Management

Stress = a positive, motivating force
Too much stress = **DISTRESS** = a harmful force

To reduce stress:

* Exercise.

* Talk to someone about worries, concerns.

* Know your limits. Set limits.

* Make time for fun.

* Know what you have to do. Do one thing at the time.

* Know it's O.K. to cry.

* Avoid self-medication.

Time Management

* Know that some time will be spent on activities beyond your control.

* Make a daily "to do" list.

* Do the most important/difficult things first.

* Save up errands to do at once.

* Take along a small task if going somewhere you know you will have to wait.

* Do an appraisal of the things you must do. Delegate ones you can. Forget unnecessary ones.

continued

Decision-Making

* Define and clarify the issue.

* Set up criteria that any solution or decision should meet. For example: there is enough time; it is affordable.

* Select the best possible solution for everybody involved.

* Design a plan of action.

Life-style Management

* Exercise.

* Eat right.

* Get enough rest.

* Take time to relax.

* Maintain a sense of humor.

* Get regular medical and dental check-ups.

* Use positive self-talk. ("I am a coper." "It may be difficult, but I can manage this.")

* Develop and use a support system.

Social Support Systems

A personal support system is made up of the individuals, agencies, and organizations with which a caregiver has direct or indirect contact.

Social support may include:

- physical or practical assistance
- resource and information sharing
- emotional and psychological assistance
- attitude transmission

Benefits of social support include:

- Reduced stress
- Decreased physical health problems
- Improved emotional well-being

Assessing *Your* Social Support Network

1. Who are the people who help you? (Circle all that apply)

   The people who help me include

Spouse	Doctor(s)	Professional agencies
Parents	Nurse(s)	public health
Children	Members of the	schools
Other relatives	congregation	social services
Pastor	Co-workers	respite care
Friends	Support group	activity programs
Other caregivers	Civic groups/clubs	

2. Identify at least one of the above who helps you in each of the following ways:
   a. Provides physical/practical assistance (example: transportation, groceries, assistance with chores)

   b. Provides resources and information (example: information on community services)

   c. Provides emotional/psychological assistance (example: listens, encourages)

   d. Provides a positive outlook/attitude (example: helps to laugh and see things more positively)

continued

3. What are some of the practical reasons we have for not using relatives, friends, and neighbors for social support and that they have for not providing support?

4. What are some beliefs and attitudes that others may have which prevent them from offering support to you?

5. What are some beliefs and attitudes you have which may be preventing you from accepting or seeking support from others?

6. What steps could you take to cope with the barriers (practical as well as attitudes and beliefs) that prevent you from getting the support you need?

Caregivers . . .

~

"Caregivers have a unique role to play in an individual's struggle with life-threatening illness. That role might be compared to a candle. A candle can help illuminate an experience, provide a path in the darkness, and give courage to explore. Caregivers, at their best, can provide that light. That light can accompany individuals as they negotiate a sometimes treacherous and scary path. The journey [may] still be dark, but the light can make it less terrifying."

Source: Doka, K. J. (1993). *Living with life-threatening illness: A guide for patients, their families and caregivers.* New York, NY: Lexington, p. 247.

Module 3
Building Cooperative Relationships

Purposes of Session

The purposes of this session are:

* to help participants recognize the importance of cooperative relationships between formal and informal caregivers.

* to introduce different styles of formal/informal caregiver relationships.

* to discuss ways of being a more helpful caregiver and building cooperative relationships.

* to introduce essential elements needed to build cooperative relationships.

* to examine skills needed to maintain cooperative relationships.

Relationship Triangle and Relationship Styles Summary

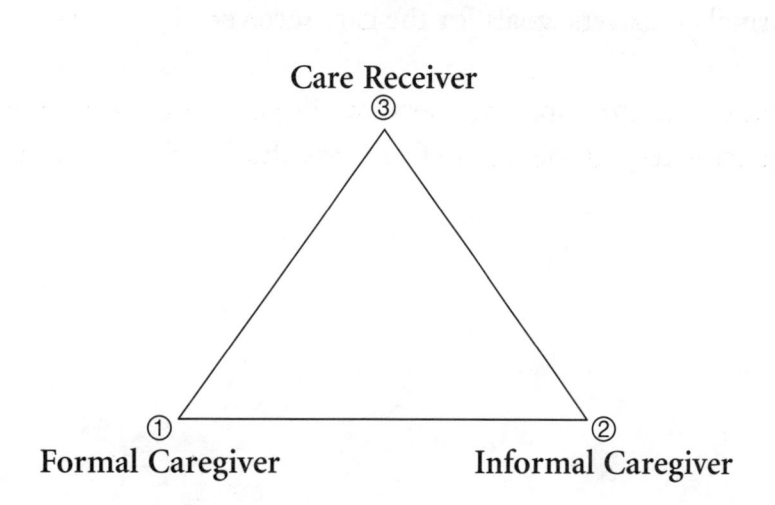

```
            Care Receiver
                 ③

                /\
               /  \
              /    \
             /      \
            /        \
           /          \
          /            \
         ①────────────②
   Formal Caregiver   Informal Caregiver
```

Relationship Styles

1. *Competitive Relationships:*
    * Interaction tends to be negative, adversarial
    * Lack of support for concerns, priorities, or efforts of the other

2. *Independent Relationships:*
    * Little interaction between formal/informal caregivers
    * Little purposeful collaboration or support for each other's concerns, priorities, or efforts on behalf of the care receiver
    * Little chance of a relationship developing
    * Random benefits to care receiver
    * Efforts of two parties are usually at cross purposes

In the above two styles of relationships, the caregivers become focused on one another and often forget about the needs of the care receiver.

3. *Cooperative Relationships:*
    * Commitment to constructive resolution of conflict
    * Commitment to collaboration (developing common goals and commitments; sharing resources and decision-making responsibilities)

continued

- Genuine interest in each other's concerns and priorities for care receiver
- Purposeful reinforcement of each other's efforts
- Greater opportunity to arrive at a plan that reflects both the formal and informal caregivers' goals for the care receiver

In this type of relationship, caregivers are cooperative collaborators; that is, they are working together to provide the best care possible for the care receiver.

How to Be a More Helpful Caregiver

Part A. For Informal Caregivers

1. Think of a formal (professional) caregiver who was particularly *unhelpful* to you. List some of the things that made him/her seem unhelpful.

2. Think of a formal (professional) caregiver who was particularly *helpful* to you. List some of the things that made him/her seem helpful.

3. Compare the characteristics of the two caregivers described above. What suggestions or "tips" could you offer formal caregivers on being more helpful?

continued

Part B. For Formal Caregivers

1. Think of an informal caregiver who you found particularly *unhelpful* in working with you. List some of the things that made him/her seem unhelpful.

2. Think of an informal caregiver who you found particularly *helpful* in working with you. List some of the things that made him/her seem helpful.

3. Compare the characteristics of the two informal caregivers described above. What suggestions or "tips" could you offer informal caregivers on being more helpful?

Building and Maintaining a Cooperative Relationship

Elements Needed for Building a Cooperative Relationship

1. **Effective communication**
   * Being open and genuine
   * Expressing oneself and listening

2. **Mutual respect**
   * Viewing each other as equal members of the caregiving team
   * Sharing ideas, information, and feelings
   * Sharing common values and experiences

3. **Trust**
   * Allowing time for this aspect of the relationship to develop

Skills Needed to Maintain a Cooperative Relationship

1. **Perspective taking**
   * Understanding the positions taken by the other persons by learning what makes them believe, feel, and behave the way they do.
   * Appreciating the good intentions that motivate caregivers

2. **Positive reinforcement**
   * Expressing appreciation
   * Offering other rewards

3. **Frequent contact**
   * Keeping up communication

Suggestions for Developing Trust and Respect Between Formal and Informal Caregivers

FORMAL

1. Accept informal caregivers as they are.

2. Listen actively to the concerns and needs expressed by informal caregivers.

3. Share all information and resources that you are legally and ethically allowed to share.

4. Prepare for all meetings with informal caregivers.

5. Keep your word. Return calls promptly and share materials as promised.

6. Allow the informal caregivers' expertise to shine.

7. Be available when needed.

INFORMAL

1. Accept formal caregivers as they are.

2. Listen actively to information and concerns shared by the formal caregiver(s).

3. Give all important information about the conditions of the care receiver and your own concerns to the formal caregiver(s).

4. Prepare for all meetings with formal caregivers.

5. Keep your word. Try not to make offers or promises you cannot keep.

6. Allow the formal caregivers' expertise to shine.

7. Make yourself available or keep formal caregiver(s) advised of your whereabouts.

MODULE 4
Preventing and Solving Problems

Purposes of Session

The purposes of this session are:

* to identify common problems faced by caregivers.

* to discuss guidelines for problem solving.

* to describe a five-step model for problem solving.

* to provide an opportunity for participants to practice using the model on a case study (as a class).

* to provide an opportunity for participants to practice using the model (in small groups) on real-life problems being faced by caregivers in this program.

Problem Solving Guidelines

Problem solving is the procedure we follow when developing plans for responding to life challenges. It is both a practical skill and a confidence builder.*

1. Understand that problem situations are a normal part of life for all of us.

2. Develop a self-perception that you are a problem solver. Keep telling yourself, "I am a problem solver."

3. Approach problem situations calmly, logically, and rationally; not impulsively, emotionally, or passively.

4. Approach problems systematically, taking one step at a time, so that they do not become overwhelming. ("Bite off small pieces.")

5. Use your available social support system in solving the problem. Don't hesitate to ask others to help in problem solving. Social support systems include family members, friends, co-workers, agencies, professional service providers and community/civic organizations.

6. Use good communication (an essential ingredient in problem solving). Share information openly and don't be afraid to ask questions.

7. Keep in mind that in most situations there is not one "correct" solution or course of action—just the best choice among available alternatives.

8. Understand that successful problem solving may not be easy. It often takes hard work and cooperation.

9. Practice your problem solving skills. They will improve dramatically with practice.

---

*From Kleinke, C. C. (1991). *Coping with life challenges.* Pacific Grove, CA: Brooks/Cole Publishing Co., p. 31.

The Ima Caregiver Situation

~

Ima Caregiver is a 77-year-old widow who lives with her 39-year-old daughter, Eura. Eura had an accident in her preteen years which left her paralyzed from the shoulders down. She must use a wheelchair for mobility and she stays at home most of the time. Her mental functioning is fine, though she is subject to occasional boredom and depression. Eura needs some medical care, but her condition is stable. She does need a great deal of assistance with personal care activities and moving from chair to bed, etc.

Ima's husband helped with some aspects of Eura's care, such as lifting and moving her when necessary, especially in his younger years. He died suddenly of a heart attack three years ago. Ima has two other children, a 45-year-old son who lives with his wife and two children approximately 100 miles away, and a 42-year-old daughter who is divorced and lives with her two youngest children about 600 miles away. (The daughter's oldest child, a daughter, is married and attends a state university about 150 miles away from Ima).

Ima has arthritis in her hands and knees. She is finding it more and more difficult to lift and move Eura. She pays a housekeeper to come in four days a week to help with cooking and cleaning. The housekeeper also helps some with the care of Eura, but Ima does not like for her to be left in complete charge of Eura's care (and neither does the housekeeper).

Ima has her own car, and is able to tend to most of her personal business. But she is concerned about her ability to continue caring for Eura as she gets older. She has several good friends with whom she visits frequently, by telephone and in person. Occasionally, she goes out with friends, but finding care for Eura is difficult. She has not been away on a "vacation" since her husband died. Some days she feels fine but on others it is a struggle to make it through the day.

Ima lives on a fixed income, and her husband's life insurance has provided well for her. Most of Eura's medical expenses are covered. Ima is able to live comfortably on the income she receives, but she has very little money in savings or investments.

Steps in Problem Solving

Step 1: Define the problem

- Try to understand exactly what is involved with the problem.
- Determine the critical issues, conflicts, and persons involved.
- Make sure you are identifying the "real" problem and not just the symptoms.
- Gather information from all relevant sources.
- State the problem in a solvable, action-oriented form. (Do not include unsolvable problems, or ones over which you have no control.)
- Include members of your social support network in identifying the problem. (They can encourage us to take an objective view and examine all sides of the problem.)
- Be specific about the problem and state it in a concise form.

Step 2: Identify and list alternative solutions

- Use a "brainstorming" technique.
- List as many options for solving the problem as possible.
- Do not evaluate or censor ideas as they are presented.
- Encourage spontaneous ideas from all participating.
- Be creative and open to exchanging ideas in a non-judgmental and non-self conscious manner.
- Make sure that everybody has a chance to give ideas and that no one dominates the process.

continued

Step 3: Evaluate options and choose a course of action

- Reduce the list of options by omitting those which are clearly not feasible or violate legal, ethical, or value concerns.
- Evaluate the usefulness of each of the remaining options.
- Consider the possible outcomes (positive and negative) of each option.
- Combine two or more individual options if this results in a better solution to the problem.
- Make other necessary improvements to the listed options.
- Select the option which appears to be the most feasible or have the best likely outcomes.
- Have an alternate plan in case the first option does not work out.

Step 4: Take action/implement the solution

- Map out a strategy for implementing the solution; plan out, step-by-step.
- Determine who will be responsible for each of the necessary tasks and make sure everyone agrees to accept his/her responsibility.
- Carry out the assigned tasks.
- Continue to maintain frequent communication.

Step 5: Test and adjust the solution

- Try out the selected course of action.
- Be open to feedback about its success from all who are involved.
- Make adjustments in implementing the plan, as necessary.
- Be prepared to try the alternate solution, or go back into the problem solving process, if the implementation plan is really not working. Also:
  —Consider any new information.
  —Select other options as appropriate.

MODULE 5
Accessing and Developing Resources

Purposes of Session

The purposes of this session are:

* to identify barriers to accessing caregiving resources in the community.

* to give participants practical guidelines and strategies for navigating the formal system of care and services.

* to present participants with resource guides, directories, and persons with information specific to their own communities.

* to assist participants in identifying and using their personal social support networks.

Basic Guidelines for Navigating the System

1. **Do your homework. Prepare before attempting to navigate the system.**

    * Gather important information about the person you are caring for (health status, insurance coverage, family financial problems and strengths, personal information).
    * Prepare in advance for meetings or conferences with professionals or specialists.
    * Learn all you can about resources for services in your area, including types of service available, admissions criteria, and service philosophy.
    * Talk with others about their experiences with agencies and individuals in the system.

2. **Prepare for the worst, but keep as positive an attitude as possible.**

    * Expect delays, wrong information, unhelpful people, and frustration.
    * Keep things in perspective and try not to be overly concerned with "minor details."
    * Try not to be overly critical of others in the system.

3. **Evaluate the potential services for the person you are caring for before committing to them.**

    * Is the service really needed?
    * Could it be provided in a more effective way?
    * What are potential benefits and risks?
    * Is it cost-effective? (worth the cost?)

4. **Whenever possible, involve the person you are caring for in decisions about the most appropriate services and keep them informed of your success and frustrations.**

continued

5. **Keep your own records of contacts and experiences with agencies, organizations, and individuals.**
    * Write down and save information and accounts of your experiences. Include dates, times, names of persons you talked with, what was said, etc.
    * Keep copies of everything: letters to and from service providers, insurance forms, etc.

6. **Use guides, forms, and gimmicks which have been developed by others to help you locate, discuss, and evaluate resources.**
    * Telephone question checklist.
    * Service evaluation checklist.
    * Questions to ask service providers.

7. **Never give up on seeking the best for the person you are helping or stop looking out for their best interests.**
    * Work through appropriate channels within the system when possible.
    * If concerns are not addressed within the system, apply pressure on the system, but consider the seriousness of your situation, the likelihood of success and possible repercussions.

8. **Be your own advocate, advocate for others, and accept advocacy from others.**
    * Speak up for yourself and the person you are caring for.
    * Enlist support from family members, friends, co-workers, professional associates or organizations.
    * Participate in an organized support group.

9. **Accept your own limitations and those of others (professionals, family members, care receiver).**

10. **When you feel that you have done all the study and preparation you can, trust your own judgment and intuition when making decisions about the care of your loved one or client.**

Caring for You, Caring for Me: Education and Support Program for Caregivers

~

Participant Evaluation

Thank you for being a participant in the *Caring for You, Caring for Me* education and support program. We need your honest feedback about this program as we revise it for future presentation. Please take a few moments to complete this evaluation form. Thank you for your comments!

Please rate the following aspects of this education and support program by placing a check (✔) in the appropriate box:

	Excellent	Good	Fair	Poor
1. Quality of Instruction				
2. Material/Information Presented				
3. Number of Sessions				
4. Length of each session				
5. Topics Covered				
6. Organization of Topics				
7. Facilities				
8. Breaks/Refreshments				
9. Overall Rating				

10. How convenient for you was the time of day at which the sessions were offered? (Check one.)
    - ☐ Very Convenient
    - ☐ Convenient
    - ☐ Somewhat Convenient
    - ☐ Not Very Convenient

continued

Would there have been a better time of day for you to attend? (Please be specific.)

The topics for the five sessions of this program were:
   a. What does it mean to be a caregiver?
   b. Taking care of yourself
   c. Building cooperative relationships
   d. Preventing and solving problems
   e. Accessing and developing resources

11. Which of these topics was *most* helpful to you? (Circle one.)

                  a   b   c   d   e

Please explain:

12. Were any of these topics **not** helpful to you? (Circle all that apply.)

                  a   b   c   d   e

Please explain:

continued

13. Are there any of these topics on which you would like to have spent more time in class? (Circle one.)

YES   NO

If YES, which one(s)?

14. What, if anything, would you change about this program?

15. How helpful was it to you to be in a group that included both formal and informal caregivers? (Check one.)
    ☐ Very Helpful
    ☐ Helpful
    ☐ Somewhat Helpful
    ☐ Not Helpful

    Comments:

16. Would you recommend this education and support program to other caregivers you know? (Circle one.)

    YES   NO

17. Are you (check all that apply):
    ☐ a formal caregiver
    ☐ an informal caregiver
    ☐ a volunteer caregiver

18. Please use the space below for any additional comments you would like to make about this program.

APPENDIX A
The Rosalynn Carter Institute

The Rosalynn Carter Institute (RCI) was established in 1987 on the campus of Georgia Southwestern State University in Americus, Georgia. The mission of the Institute is to understand the process of caregiving and discover new ways to benefit both formal and informal caregivers for persons with emotional and mental problems, difficulties of the frail elderly, developmental disabilities or physical illnesses. The RCI conducts research on the caregiving process; provides educational programs for caregivers; consults with agencies and organizations on caregiving issues; provides a forum for discussion of issues concerning formal and informal caregivers; disseminates information on caregiving to a wide audience; and advocates for public awareness and policy changes which enhance the lives of caregivers.

The Rosalynn Carter Institute believes that, while caregiving is rewarding, it also produces circumstances which may jeopardize the psychological well-being of those providing care and, when caregivers suffer, the quality of care they are able to provide is diminished. On the other hand, if caregivers are supported and maintain their own emotional and physical health, the well-being of the person receiving care will ultimately be enhanced. The Rosalynn Carter Institute also supports the notion that caregivers and care receivers can be served most effectively through the collaborative efforts of formal and informal caregivers, academicians, public and private services, and organizations representing caregivers and recipients of care.

The mission of the Institute is implemented primarily through two major initiatives—one regional and the other national. The West Central Georgia Caregivers' Network (CARE-NET) addresses concerns of informal and formal caregivers in a sixteen-county region of Georgia. The CARE-NET is governed by its Leadership Council composed of distinguished formal and informal caregivers in the region, including persons in leadership positions with various agencies and organizations. The network promotes opportunities for linking formal and informal caregivers throughout the region in collaborative endeavors; oversees research conducted by the RCI; develops service and educational programs to meet the needs of caregivers; and provides recognition and support of caregivers. In conjunction with the CARE-NET, the Rosalynn

Carter Institute conducted an extensive study of formal and informal caregivers in the west central Georgia region. In 1993, the RCI published and disseminated the results in a report entitled *Characteristics, Concerns, and Concrete Needs of Formal and Informal Caregivers: Understanding and Appreciating their Marathon Existence* (Nottingham, et al., 1993). The needs and concerns of caregivers reported in this study formed the basis for future directions of the CARE-NET and the RCI. In 1997, a second CARE-NET, the South Georgia Caregivers Network, was created in conjunction with the Division of Social Work at Valdosta State University.

The National Quality Caregiving Coalition (NQCC) is composed of national associations and organizations representing formal and informal caregivers and recipients of care. The mission of the NQCC is to explore the nature of quality caregiving; promote public recognition of the value of caregiving and the contributions of caregivers; and facilitate the development of a true partnership between formal and informal caregivers and recipients of care, in an atmosphere of compassion, collaboration and respect.

APPENDIX B
Suggested Readings for Formal and Informal Caregivers

∽

The list of suggested readings which is contained in this appendix was prepared by the Rosalynn Carter Institute to assist both informal and formal caregivers in gaining more in-depth knowledge to assist them in their caregiving roles. The listing for each book contains the author(s), year of publication, title, publisher, number of pages, and a brief description. The list is arranged into topics according to the various health situations creating the need for care. These topics are presented in alphabetical order. Within each topic, books are listed in alphabetical order according to author. Resources marked with an asterisk (*) were written for professionally trained caregivers such as physicians, nurses, psychologists, social workers and counselors.

This reading list does not include all books which have been written about caregiving. It is a listing of books which have been reviewed by staff of the Rosalynn Carter Institute and considered potentially helpful to formal or informal caregivers. Each year, many new books about caregiving are published and it is virtually impossible to have an updated listing of such books. You are encouraged to ask your program leader, local librarians, or representatives of caregiving organizations for their recommendations of additional books which may be beneficial to caregivers.

Contents

AIDS   53

Alzheimer's Disease and Related Disorders   53

Books for Children   55
    Attention Deficit Hyperactivity Disorder   55
    Cancer   55
    Cerebral Palsy   55
    Diabetes   55
    Down Syndrome   55
    Epilepsy   55
    General Topics   56
    Mental Illness   56

Cancer   56

Care of Elderly   57

Care of Terminally Ill   61

Children with Special Needs   61
    Attention Deficit Hyperactivity Disorder   61
    Autism   61
    Cerebral Palsy   62
    Down Syndrome   63
    Epilepsy   63
    General Topics   63
    Mental Retardation   65

Chronic Illness   66

Congregational Caregiving   67

Coping and Self-Care for the Caregiver   67

Diabetes   69

Eating Disorders   70

Elderly as Caregivers   70

General Topics   70

Loss and Grief   76

Mental Illness   77
    Depression   77
    General Topics   78
    Schizophrenia   79

Multiple Sclerosis   79

Parkinson's Disease   80

Planning for the Future (Financial, Legal, Educational, etc.)   80

Stroke   81

Support/Self-Help Groups   81

AIDS

Garfield, Charles (1995). *Sometimes my heart goes numb: Love and caregiving in a time of AIDS.* San Francisco, CA: Jossey-Bass. (298 pgs).

> This book offers portraits of twenty caregivers of persons with HIV/AIDS. It also reveals the risks and rewards of giving care to a person with a chronic or life-threatening illness. Some of the topics discussed are: active listening; coping with losses; bereavement; saying the right thing; and taking care of oneself while giving care to others.

*Landau-Stanton, Judith (1993). *AIDS, health and mental health.* New York: Brunner/Mazel. (343 pgs).

> The authors of this book are concerned with assisting professionals to become better educated concerning the AIDS virus. Discussions include correcting AIDS myths, systems impacted by AIDS, populations at risk, health care providers at risk, and clinical management of AIDS.

Alzheimer's Disease and Related Disorders

Bridges, Barbara J. (1995). *Therapeutic caregiving: A practical guide for caregivers of persons with Alzheimer's and other dementia causing diseases.* Mill Creek, WA: BJB Publishing. (214 pgs).

> *Therapeutic caregiving* offers professional expertise and practical advice. The author presents techniques for keeping people with dementia more functional physically and mentally. How to maintain adequate nutrition and oral hygiene, assist with bathing and dressing, help with exercise, manage behavior problems, and deal with confusion and depression are only some of the topics covered. Both long-term care professionals and family members can benefit from the practical suggestions and pictured exercises. Caregivers dealing with people who have strokes, Parkinson's disease, etc. would also benefit from this manual.

Coughlan, Patricia B. (1993). *Facing Alzheimer's: Family caregivers speak.* New York, NY: Ballantine Books. (261 pgs).

> When the body and mind of a loved one begin to fail, the burden that falls on the caregiver can be overwhelming. In this deeply practical and warmhearted book, eight women who lived through their husbands' declines talk frankly about how they faced the agonizing decisions they had to make and live with, including acknowledging the illness, adjusting to profound changes in one's spouse, coping with crisis, nurturing one's own sanity and health, and preparing for the end and a new beginning.

Danforth, Art (1984). *Living with Alzheimer's: Ruth's story.* Falls Church, VA: Prestige Press. (219 pgs).

> *Living with Alzheimer's: Ruth's story* is the moving and heartwarming story of the life shared by two victims of dementia: Art's wife, Ruth, whose mental deterioration he lived with every day for seven years and Art, the caregiver. Art shares with the reader not only his love for Ruth and his fears for her safety, but also his anger and sense of guilt.

Doernberg, Myrna (1986). *Stolen mind: The slow disappearance of Ray Doernberg.* Chapel Hill, NC: Algonquin Books. (223 pgs).

> A wife vividly tells the story of her husband's progressive dementia; what she, her husband, and their two sons experienced dealing with his disease; and the many ways this disaster affected their family.

Dwyer, Sharon A. R., Sloane, Phillip D., & Barrick, Ann Louise (1995). *Solving bathing problems in persons with Alzheimer's disease and related dementias: A training and reference manual for caregivers.* Chapel Hill, NC: University of North Carolina. (68 pgs).

> The authors provide answers to commonly asked questions about problems related to bathing persons with dementia. General guidelines for bathing persons with dementia and procedures for dealing with specific bathing problems are included. Also explained are methods for developing a personal hygiene care plan and maintaining the quality of bathing procedures.

Feil, Naomi (1993). *The validation breakthrough: Simple techniques for communicating with people with "Alzheimer's-type dementia."* Baltimore, MD: Health Professions Press. (320 pgs).

> Validation therapy is a tool to aid in the communication with people who have Alzheimer's-type dementia. It shows caregivers how they can reduce conflict and stress by validating feelings rather than focusing on confusion. The author explains specifically how to use validation therapy with individuals who are maloriented, time confused, repetitive movers, etc.

Gruetzner, Howard (1992). *Alzheimer's: A caregiver's guide and sourcebook.* New York, NY: John Wiley & Sons. (310 pgs).

> This guide leads the reader through the realities of caring for and coping with a person with Alzheimer's disease. The latest developments in treatment and care options are detailed. Topics covered include: the symptoms and traits of Alzheimer's, what to expect at each progressive stage, how to respond to behavior problems, the full range of treatments and supportive services available, suggestions on managing personal stress, the importance of the family in the successful care of Alzheimer's patients, and ways to understand feelings and the impact of grief. The author shows caregivers how to make the care they give more rewarding and more effective, and the life of the patient safer and more comfortable.

Heston, Leonard L., & White, June A. (1991). *The vanishing mind: A practical guide to Alzheimer's disease and other dementias.* New York, NY: W. H. Freeman. (191 pgs)

> The authors of this guide offer specific and detailed information on dementia, and various diseases that result in a condition of dementia. Chapters explore topics including signs and symptoms of dementia, diseases that cause dementia, specialists and tests, medical treatment and management of dementia, care alternatives, and practical matters such as children, neighbors, finances, and insurance.

Mace, Nancy L. (1990). *Dementia care: Patient, family, and community.* Baltimore, MD: Johns Hopkins University Press. (400 pgs)

> This sourcebook covers a wealth of information on dementia care, including the diagnostic assessment of patients, their clinical care, management of behavior problems, therapeutic activity, and issues in late-stage care. The family is considered in discussions of support, home environment, respite care, and financial and legal considerations. Long-term care services, volunteer programs, residential care and public policy are explored.

Murphy, Beverly Bigtree (1995). *He used to be somebody: A journey into Alzheimer's disease through the eyes of a caregiver.* Boulder, CO: Gibbs Associates. (348 pgs).

> This author gives a first-hand account of the onset of Alzheimer's disease through its progression into the final stages. Murphy has a unique view of this illness from professional and personal standpoints, resulting in her ability to offer practical, first-hand insights on subjects such as adapting the home, handling incontinence, dealing with the behavior changes, and grief and mourning. The author/caregiver shares the sense of isolation, fear, loss, and continuous state of mourning one goes through when losing a loved one to a progressive, degenerative disease. A unique feature of this book is the inclusion of the reprinted words of famous songs which poignantly illustrate the significant stages of Alzheimer's disease and the feelings of the people involved with the illness during each of these stages.

Roberts, D. Jeanne (1991). *Taking care of caregivers: For families and others who care for people with Alzheimer's disease and other forms of dementia.* Palo Alto, CA: Bull Publishing. (181 pgs).

> *Taking care of caregivers* inspires and empowers caregivers so that they can maintain their own health, happiness, and sanity in order to provide loving care for the person who is ill. With descriptions of the problems and exercises to help find solutions, this guide covers many important topics including: the needs of caregivers, communication and feelings, grief and its various phases, sharing and support, and stress management techniques.

*Wright, Lore K. (1993). *Alzheimer's disease and marriage: An intimate account.* Newbury Park, CA: Sage. (147 pgs).

> *Alzheimer's disease and marriage* peers into caregiving research and personal data on individual

relationships to uncover the profound effects of Alzheimer's disease on marriage. The author shows how the disease invades various dimensions of marriage and how spouses retain or lose awareness of each other. Among the marital dimensions explored are day-to-day aspects of a relationship, such as household tasks, tension, companionship, affection and sexuality, and commitment. Clinical assessment strategies and guidelines for interventions are described. Details on how to approach and interact with an affected spouse are also provided.

Books for Children

Attention Deficit Hyperactivity Disorder

Quinn, Patricia O., & Stern, Judith M. (1991). *Putting on the brakes: Young people's guide to understanding Attention Deficit Hyperactivity Disorder.* New York, NY: Magination Press.

> This down-to-earth, upbeat guide contains a wealth of information and practical suggestions for coping with the problems that Attention Deficit Hyperactivity Disorder (ADHD) presents. The authors explore the nature and treatment of ADHD, as well as gaining control, getting support, and making friends. Quinn and Stern's purpose is to give kids a sense of control and a perception of obtainable goals.

Cancer

Trillin, Alice (1996). *Dear Bruno.* New York, NY: The New Press. (32 pgs).

> This book is written for children who have cancer (or other serious illnesses) by a woman who previously had cancer and recovered. It is written as a letter which discusses the ill person's experiences with physicians, hospitals, and what it is like to have a serious illness. This book is nicely illustrated by Edward Koren and has a foreword by Paul Newman.

Cerebral Palsy

Grimm, Eric (no date). *Walk with me.* Washington, DC: United Cerebral Palsy Association. (50 pgs).

> *Walk with me* is a touching story, written by an eight-year-old boy with cerebral palsy. In it, Eric tells what it's like to be a child facing this disability, and the feelings that he experiences. Included is a checklist of strategies to use when communicating with a person who has a disability. This book is excellent reading for children who interact with a child with cerebral palsy, either at school or at home.

Diabetes

Mulder, Linnea (1992). *Sarah and Puffle: A story for children about diabetes.* New York, NY: Magination Press.

> A stuffed sheep comes to life just in time to help a young girl who is feeling angry and sad because she has diabetes. Puffle's funny rhymes are full of valuable advice sure to comfort all children with diabetes, and to further understanding by siblings and friends. Parents will appreciate the clearly written introduction.

Down Syndrome

Berkus, Clara W. (1992). *Charlsie's chuckle.* Rockville, MD: Woodbine House. (32 pgs).

> This is the story of an adventurous seven-year-old boy with Down Syndrome who becomes the local hero when his laugh brings harmony to his hometown. On his birthday, Charlsie gets a bicycle and takes off on a special adventure. This book teaches that every child can make a significant contribution, and that a little laughter can make a big difference.

Epilepsy

Moss, Deborah M. (1989). *Lee: The rabbit with epilepsy.* Kensington, MD: Woodbine House. (12 pgs).

> The imaginative tale of Lee and her family explains epilepsy in a manner that children can easily understand. Lee's epilepsy is followed from her first seizure through her diagnosis and treatment. The author takes a compassionate, yet realistic view of epilepsy. The book is a valuable guide for a child with epilepsy as well as the sibling or friend of one. The message is one of hope and understanding regarding children with disabilities.

General Topics

Kriegsman, Kay H., Zaslow, Elinor L., & O'Zmura-Rechsteiner, Jennifer (1992). *Taking charge: Teenagers talk about life and physical disabilities.* Rockville, MD: Woodbine House. (164 pgs).

> *Taking charge* delivers honest advice on a wide range of issues that teens with physical disabilities face during adolescence. This book covers three major areas of concern: Part one focuses on the individual and self-esteem; part two explores relationships with friends, family, and the community; and part three looks toward the future with a discussion of long- and short-term goals and how to achieve them. Appendices include a wealth of useful information.

Mills, Joyce C. (1992). *Little tree: A story for children with serious medical problems.* New York, NY: Magination Press.

> This sensitive story addresses the emotional difficulties of a child with a serious illness, and offers a powerful healing metaphor that the child will remember after the book is closed. Medical procedures are subtly and symbolically mirrored with messages of hope and healing.

Peterken, Allan. (1992). *What about me?* New York, NY: Magination Press. (Unpaged).

> When children become seriously ill, their brothers and sisters are often confused and experience conflicting emotions. Children will identify with Laura, a young girl with a sick brother, who experiences the normal feelings of confusion, guilt, anger, and isolation when her parents seem to spend all their time at the hospital, and all the attention is focused on her ill brother. Children reading this story will see their feelings being acknowledged and can gain a greater understanding of their situation.

Powell, Thomas H., & Gallagher, Peggy A. (1993). *Brothers and sisters: A special part of exceptional families.* Baltimore, MD: Paul H. Brookes. (289 pgs).

> Rich with personal testimonies, this compelling book shares the joys and sorrows so familiar to exceptional families. Siblings speak openly about the challenges they encounter in interactions with their brothers or sisters, and discuss how these interactions affect them in all aspects of their lives. Brimming with practical advice, this guide also includes a list of 30 parental strategies and 20 sibling strategies suggested by a panel of siblings.

Thompson, Mary (1992). *My brother, Matthew.* Rockville, MD: Woodbine House.

> Siblings of children with disabilities often have trouble adjusting and have feelings of being "left out." In this tale, David has a younger brother born with disabilities. He tells what happens in his family and what it's like to be Matthew's brother. Siblings' normal feelings of loneliness, rejection, and impatience are addressed, along with a message of hope and understanding.

Mental Illness

Lanskin, Pamela L., & Moskowitz, Addie A. (1991). *Wish upon a star: A story for children with a parent who is mentally ill.* New York, NY: Magination Press.

> Children of a parent with mental illness often feel confused, frightened, lonely, and ashamed. In this poignant tale, a little girl expresses her confusion over the behavior of her mother who has a mental illness, and the hurt she feels when her mother doesn't seem to pay attention to her anymore. Children will be comforted by having their feelings described, and others will gain a greater appreciation for the difficulty these children face.

Cancer

Benjamin, Harold H. (1995). *The wellness community: Guide to fighting for recovery from cancer.* New York, NY: G.P. Putnam's Sons. (270 pgs).

> This book contains many insightful ideas and a great deal of information about fighting for recovery from cancer. Topics include: fighting for one's recovery; how to control stress; how to use directed visualization; how to regain hope, take back control, and reduce anger; common questions people with cancer ask; what the Wellness Community is and the services it provides; the Wellness Community nutrition guide; and a list of The Wellness Community facilities and additional resources.

Gee, Elizabeth D. (1992). *The light around the dark.* Hudson Street, NY: National League for Nursing Press. (150 pgs).

The Light Around the Dark tells Elizabeth Gee's story of caring, of her life of living her ethics, and of her humanity. It tells a story of suffering and triumph, of despair and joys, and of accomplishments. In this work, anyone who has been touched by the complex experiences associated with cancer will be lifted up by the peace and strength she found throughout her life. Readers will be encouraged by her victorious struggles with living and dying, with being connected, being alone, mothering, spousing—in being all she could be.

Rosenblum, Daniel (1993). *A time to hear, a time to help: Listening to people with cancer.* New York, NY: Free Press. (289 pgs).

Dr. Rosenblum, drawing on his long experience as a leading oncologist, shows that the greatest assistance friends, relatives, and even the physicians of people with cancer can offer is to treat them as full human beings with dignity and respect, rather than as "cancer patients." He points out that the most thoughtful and most comforting thing one can do many times is to just listen. *A time to hear, a time to help* is a personal testimony to the often difficult and painful process of learning how to listen. Through intimate portraits, Rosenblum teaches readers to understand the problems people with cancer and their caregivers face (anxiety, anger, denial, loss of self-esteem, facing death, etc.), and the importance of compassion, patience, and understanding in offering comfort to them.

Care of Elderly

*Barresi, Charles M. (1993). *Ethnic elderly and long term care.* New York: Springer. (289 pgs).

Barresi gives a professional overview of the special needs of ethnic elderly persons. He explores ethnic variations in measurement of physical health; minority issues in family caregiving; Black and Hispanic caregivers of dementia victims; self care practices of Black elders; institutional care in ethnic settings; models of ethnically sensitive care; and planning, policy and practice.

*Biegel, David E. (1990). *Aging and caregiving.* Newbury Park, CA: Sage. (294 pgs).

This book thoroughly covers research conducted in the area of aging and caregiving dealing with theory and methodology, cognitive and physical impairment, and public policy perspectives. Some of the specific topics covered are: the psychological impact of caregiving on the caregiver; ethical issues in a family caregiving situation; stress of caregivers; and women as caregivers of the elderly.

*Cantor, Marjorie H. (Ed.). (1994). *Family caregiving: Agenda for the future.* San Francisco, CA: American Society on Aging. (149 pgs).

This book of readings contains papers presented at the 1993 Critical Issues Forum conducted by the American Society on Aging. Family caregiving is discussed from a number of angles, including research and personal perspectives, public policy agenda, and training with education. Also explored are the impacts of social services and ethical, legal, and financial issues on caregivers.

Carlin, Vivian F., & Greenburg, Vivian E. (1992). *Should mom live with us? And is happiness possible if she does?* New York, NY: Lexington Books. (195 pgs)

With rising costs of care, elderly people often find themselves dependent on their adult children for a place to live and for personal care. This guide is designed to help middle-aged children and their aging parents weigh all options and make good decisions about living together. With warmth and humor, the authors explore pros and cons, discuss alternatives, then provide a blueprint for making it work.

Cohen, Donna, & Eisdorfer, Carl (1993). *Seven steps to effective parent care: A planning and action guide for adult children and their aging parents.* New York, NY: G. P. Putnam's Sons. (261 pgs).

Based on years of research and work with families, this book presents a coherent approach for caregiving that reframes aging and parent care as a process of problem solving to be managed by the entire family. The authors have segmented caregiving into small, easily accomplished steps and procedures that can substantially help in avoiding crises and family battles and eliminating many of the frustrations and fears that often accompany caring for an aging parent. Case histories are used to illustrate points. Complete listings of national and state agencies and social services involved in gerontology, mental health, and related areas are also included. Self help exercises help readers evaluate their situations.

*Decalmer, Peter, & Glendenning, Frank (Eds.). (1993). *The mistreatment of elderly people.* Newbury Park, CA: Sage. (192 pgs).

The mistreatment of elderly people argues for clearer explanations of elder abuse which go beyond immediate practical considerations and observations, and gives clear guidelines for tackling and preventing the problem. The authors include discussions of key topics such as legal implications of abuse and neglect, issues for professionals dealing with elder abuse, approaches for dealing with abuse, and models for prevention of abuse.

*Estes, Carroll L., & Swan, James H. (1993). *The long term care crisis: Elders trapped in the no-care zone.* Newbury Park, CA: Sage. (328 pgs).

The authors discuss the Prospective Payment System (PPS) for Medicare hospital reimbursement that was begun in 1984 and demonstrate its negative effects, especially on the elderly. They identify the failing of PPS and provide policy options to modify or replace it with a system that would foster greater equity in providing health care in America.

Fradkin, Louise G., & Heath, Angela (1992). *Caregiving of older adults.* Santa Barbara, CA: ABC-CLIO. (250 pgs).

In *Caregiving of older adults,* readers will find information on types of caregivers and supports, financial and legal issues, safety and welfare, housing options, and nursing home placement. One chapter is dedicated to understanding the care receiver. Also included is a valuable list of resources.

Greenberg, Vivian E. (1994). *Children of a certain age: Adults and their aging parents.* New York, NY: Lexington Books. (183 pgs).

In *Children of a certain age,* Greenberg reveals ways adult children and their aging parents can develop a mature, caring relationship based on mutual respect, trust and friendship. She explains that parenthood is always in a state of change and growth, and that parents who are open and responsive to their children not only learn from them, but will feel rejuvenated rather than frustrated and left behind. This guide shows how this can be a time to change, heal old wounds, resolve conflicts, and touch each other with affection and understanding.

Greenberg, V. E. (1989). *Your best is good enough: Aging parents and your emotions.* New York, NY: Lexington.

Time-proven strategies for coping with the conflicts and stresses inherent in caring for elderly parents are provided. With insight and skill, Vivian Greenberg offers valuable information on the needs of the elderly, the vital role emotional involvement plays in caregiving, and the need for assertive and honest communication with one's parents. She explains how to realize and accept the limits of what one can do for his/her parents; how to determine unrealistic expectations; how to get brothers and sisters to share responsibilities; and how to cope with a difficult parent. Personal anecdotes and real-life cases make this compassionate guide important reading for those who must oversee the well-being of their parents while trying to preserve their own. An appendix containing information on available resources is included.

*Gubrium, Jaber F. (1993). *Speaking of life: Horizons of meaning for nursing home residents.* Hawthorne, NY: Aldine De Gruyter. (197 pgs).

The author uses data drawn from interviews with long-term nursing home residents to explore the quality of their care and the resulting quality of their lives. These stories reveal to readers the diversity of people living in nursing homes, their views of family, their feelings of dependence/independence, their experiences of isolation and sense of self-esteem, and how they perceive the quality of their lives in nursing homes. The result is a wide variety of stories and information with valuable conceptual, methodological, and personal lessons.

*Horn, Barbara J. (1990). *Facilitating self care practices in the elderly.* Binghamton, NY: Haworth. (185 pgs).

This professional guide covers several aspects of care practices in the elderly. Horn discusses medication regimens, compliance, adverse drug reactions, the Comprehensive Medication Assessment Interview guide, tailoring teaching to the elderly in home care, and family coping with caring for the elderly.

*Kane, Rosalie A., & Penrod, Joan D. (Eds.). (1995). *Family caregiving in an aging society: Policy perspectives.* Thousand Oaks, CA: Sage. (202 pgs).

>This book considers the ramifications of the U.S. caregiving policy describing and evaluating many of the current services: respite care, individual and group therapy, and educational interventions. Topics include: prospects for family caregiving, examining respite care, direct services for family caregivers, legal and ethical issues in family caregiving and a caregiving policy for the aging family.

Koch, Tom (1993). *A place in time: Care givers for their elderly.* Westport, CT: Praeger. (236 pgs).

>*A place in time* tells the personal stories of normal people who have chosen to care for their aging and fragile relatives at home. The author uses their stories to ask: What can we learn from the experiences of others? He provides vital and practical information for anyone considering physically caring for another. Appropriate for professional and lay readers.

*Kosberg, Jordan I. (Ed.). (1992). *Family care of the elderly: Social and cultural changes.* Newbury Park, CA: Sage. (317 pgs).

>The focus of this book is on family care of the elderly in 16 different countries of the world including the United States. Every author addressed each of the following areas in discussing elder care in his/her country: traditional characteristics of the country; societal changes occurring over time; consequences of societal changes; responses to the changes in the country; and future predictions for the care of the elderly by the family and by formal service systems in the country.

Levin, Nora Jean (1993). *How to care for your parents: A handbook for adult children.* Friday Harbor, WA: Storm King Press. (110 pgs).

>This brief handbook tells readers what to expect in elder care. It includes information on the kind of decisions that will need to be made, the practical and emotional pitfalls that can occur, and on how to juggle the sometimes conflicting obligations to oneself, one's family, and one's parents. The author uses a 28-step program including time management, finances, home safety, and how best to help seniors in need.

McGurn, Sheelagh (1992). *Under one roof: Caring for an aging parent.* Park Ridge, IL: Parkside Publishing. (174 pgs). [Now available for purchase from Under One Roof, P.O. Box 9131, Mt. Prospect, IL 60056.]

>In this book, Sheelagh McGurn speaks to the increasing number of people in the "sandwich generation": those who are now taking care of both their young families and their aging parents. Many of these people are overwhelmed trying to effectively fulfill their roles as spouse, parent and caregiver. Finding doctors, arranging home health care, and coping with loved ones whose physical, mental and emotional health may be failing all add to the normal stresses of working and raising a family. Through personal experiences and interviews, McGurn addresses the day-to-day problems of caregivers and offers them both daily coping strategies and hope for the future.

Nelson-Morrill, Creston (Ed.). (1993). *Florida caregiver's handbook: An essential resource guide for caregivers and their older loved ones* (2nd ed.). Tallahassee, FL: HealthTrac Books. (272 pgs).

>This handbook covers a wide range of topics important to caregivers including: the impact of caregiving on caregivers and their families and on caregivers employed outside the home, long-distance caregiving, loss and grief, dementia, medication management, changes that may occur in the elderly as part of the normal aging process, alcohol and substance abuse, legal considerations, financial planning, nursing home decisions, dealing with the system, Medicare and Medicaid, and advocating for the care receiver. An extensive listing of elder services and caregiver support organizations with addresses and phone numbers is included. (This manual is especially written for Florida, but much of the material is helpful to people living in other states.)

*Ory, Marcia G., & Duncker, Alfred P. (Eds.). (1992). *In-home care for older people: Health and supportive services.* Newbury Park, CA: Sage. (214 pgs).

>The purpose of this book is to summarize what is known about home care for the elderly and to iden-

tify a research agenda that highlights (a) the use of in-home services for older people with different functional needs, (b) the effectiveness of different types or packages of services for different populations, and (c) the coordination of in-home services with traditional medical services. The focus is on older people in need of long-term care. The significant contribution made by family and friends and the burdens that families experience in providing care are recognized.

*Pritchard, Jacki (1992). *The abuse of elderly people: A handbook for professionals.* Philadelphia, PA: Jessica Kingsley Publishers. (174 pgs).

The abuse of elderly people is a resource and manual for the variety of professionals who work with elderly people. The four main aims of the book are: 1) to define elder abuse; 2) to raise the consciousness about elder abuse; 3) to develop skills in recognizing elder abuse; 4) to develop ways of dealing with elder abuse. The handbook provides a range of scenarios and exercises dealing with each of these areas.

Rob, Caroline (1991). *The caregiver's guide: Helping elderly relatives cope with health and safety problems.* Boston: Houghton Mifflin Company. (458 pgs).

Sensible, basic information is provided to assist in: handling medical emergencies for the elderly, recognizing both physical and mental problems, working with the latest medical advances for chronic disorders, keeping elders independent longer, and locating social services. This book is for those who are stepping in to help an older relative or friend who can no longer grapple alone with medical problems and daily living arrangements. Every section of the book is full of accessible, up-to-the-minute information about physical and emotional health. The chapters of *The caregiver's guide* are organized by conditions common in older people. The final chapter is a useful guide to accessing the social service system and network of support in communities around the country.

*Safford, Florence, & Krell, George I. (Eds.). (1992). *Gerontology for health professionals: A practice guide.* Washington, DC: National Association of Social Workers (NASW). (183 pgs).

This book provides basic principles of a humanistic perspective in health care for all professionals, but its emphasis is on providing care for the elderly which recognizes humane values, and asserts the dignity and worth of every care receiver. Topics include: understanding the experience of aging; helping the incontinent; medication; differential assessment of dementia and depression; case management with the elderly; working with traditional and nontraditional families; ethical issues; death, bereavement, loss and growth; and the impact of the elderly on the health care system with implications for the delivery of social services.

Salamon, Michael J., & Rosenthal, Gloria (1990). *Home or the nursing home: Making the right choices.* New York: Springer Publishing. (112 pgs).

The authors of this guide provide extensive information for caregivers trying to make the difficult decision between home care and nursing home care. Discussions include critical topics such as health care needs of elderly, life satisfaction, health care environments, bias/reality of nursing home vs. home care, elders and families' reactions to nursing home care and guidelines for selecting a nursing home.

Silverstone, Barbara, & Hyman, Helen K. (1992). *Growing older together: A couple's guide to understanding and coping with the challenges of later life.* New York, NY: Pantheon Books. (344 pgs).

This thoughtful and empathetic guide offers sensible, easy-to-follow advice on a variety of topics including the first signals of advancing age, retirement preparation, relationships between aging parents and their aging children, changing roles within a long-established relationship, and preserving autonomy when illness strikes. Also included are resource lists of supplementary reading, family service associations, and home-care agencies.

Smith, Kerri S. (1992). *Caring for your aging parents.* San Louis Obispo, CA: Impact Publishers. (117 pgs).

Working caregivers need a roadmap through the often confusing caregiving wilderness. *Caring for your aging parents* provides just that. It gives quick and effective solutions to common caregiving concerns including: how to make your parents' home safer and more convenient; where to find free and low cost help; how to reconcile work responsibilities with caregiving duties; how to put parent's legal and financial affairs in order; how to recognize potential medical problems; and how to regain your physical, mental, and emotional equilibrium.

Susik, D. Helen (1995). *Hiring home caregivers: The family guide to in-home eldercare.* San Luis Obispo, CA: American Source Books. (205 pgs).

This is an excellent resource guide for people who employ an in-home care helper. Topics include: the role and cost of home caregivers, selecting and hiring, background checks, supervising a helper, dealing with taxes, insurance, laws, and agency-directed home care. The lengthy and helpful appendices include tax information, publications, the IRS "tele-tax" information system, Eldercare locator, agencies on aging, and state organizations on aging.

Tuites, Ann (1995). *From grandma with love.* Lancaster, PA: Starburst. (158 pgs).

This small book offers practical emotional and spiritual support to people providing care to aging relatives. It aims to create peace, love and harmony between the generations. With entries much like a journal, the author discusses such ideas as: expectations, it's never too late to change, worrying about aging and dementia, encouragement, anger, relinquishing parental power, avoiding overprotection, and building self-esteem.

*Trieshmann, Roberta B. (1987). *Aging with a disability.* New York, NY: Demos Publications. (148 pgs).

This volume offers case studies and interviews on the topics of health, rehabilitation, and adjustment processes of older adults with disabilities. Discussion of psychosocial and environmental impacts of aging and methodological issues in aging and disability research offer valuable information for the professional interested in further research in this field.

*Young, Rosalie F. (1991). *Health, illness and disability in later life.* Newbury Park, CA: Sage. (183 pgs).

This book is a collection of essays dealing with health, illness, and disability. Essays cover topics such as status, behaviors, and risks of the elderly, health problems and family care, and the multidisciplinary aspects of health, illness, and disability in later life.

Care of Terminally Ill

Sankar, Andrea (1991). *Dying at home: A family guide for caregiving.* Baltimore, MD: Johns Hopkins Press. (257 pgs).

This book, based on interviews with family members, professional caregivers, and care receivers, discusses the decision of whether or not to provide care at home for someone who is dying. The author believes the most important reason for dying at home is that it gives the people involved as much control as possible over the process of dying. Some of the topics discussed are: preparing the home, maintaining communication with professional health care providers, maintaining the dignity of the person who is dying, financial resources, signs of approaching death, the funeral, Hospice, ethical dilemmas, caregivers taking care of themselves, and grief.

Children with Special Needs

Attention Deficit Hyperactivity Disorder

Wodrich, David L. (1994). *Attention deficit hyperactivity disorder: What every parent wants to know.* Baltimore, MD: Paul H. Brookes. (291 pgs).

Through detailed explanations, helpful checklists, and case examples, this book combines Wodrich's professional expertise with a personal sensitivity developed from working closely with the families of children with attention deficit hyperactivity disorder (ADHD). This book will help prepare parents with children suffering from ADHD for the challenges facing them at home and school and for the many decisions they will have to make about intervention and education.

Autism

Hart, Charles A. (1993). *A parent's guide to autism: Answers to the most common questions.* New York, NY: Pocket Books. (244 pgs).

Using a question-and-answer format, Hart presents information about autism and the people who have it. Included in the book is information on causes, symptoms, types of autism, diets, exercises, possible therapies and treatments, facilitated communication, and planning for the future. A resource list of books and organizations is also included.

Powers, Michael D. (1989). *Children with autism.* Rockville, MD: Woodbine House. (368 pgs).

The autistic child appears to exist in an isolated world, impossible to reach. For a parent to overcome the fears such a condition naturally arouses, he or she needs a great deal of information and hope. Powers attempts to meet this need with this comprehensive guide. From a clear description of autism, its problems, treatments, and effect on the family, to a discussion of legal rights, the author offers clear explanations with sensitivity and skill. The condition is explored from infancy to adulthood, including a discussion of residential programs and other options for adults with autism. A glossary of important terms, a reading list, and a resource guide are included.

Shulze, Craig B. (1993). *When snow turns to rain: One family's struggle to solve the riddle of autism.* Rockville, MD: Woodbine House. (216 pgs).

When snow turns to rain is a father's moving account of his family's experience with autism. Shulze recounts his personal struggle to accept and understand his son's autism, and his determination to help his child through an array of treatment and educational programs. This book affirms the strength of the human spirit, and attests to the needs of a family raising a child with a developmental disability.

Stehli, Annabel (1991). *The sound of a miracle.* New York, NY: Avon Books. (241 pgs).

The sound of a miracle is written by a mother who struggled to help her daughter, Georgie, who was diagnosed with autism. Ms. Stehli refused institutionalization as many experts and friends recommended, and sought education and treatment for her child. A new treatment for autism—auditory training—is discussed. [For detailed discussion of the auditory training, see *Hearing equals behavior* by Guy Bérard listed in "General Topics" section.]

Cerebral Palsy

Finnie, Nancie R. (1975). *Handling the young cerebral palsied child at home.* New York, NY: E. P. Dutton. (337 pgs).

This is an indispensable guide for parents, nurses, therapists, doctors, and others caring for young children with cerebral palsy. The author includes a guide to community resources and suppliers of accessories and equipment as well as detailed suggestions for supplementing a treatment program by integrating training procedures. Especially helpful for new parents are sections on abnormal postures and movements and problems parents have with handling and daily care.

Geralis, Elaine (1991). *Children with cerebral palsy: A parent's guide.* Rockville, MD: Woodbine House. (434 pgs).

This volume is essential reading for parents who want to learn about cerebral palsy and its impact on their child and family. Highly stressed is the importance of the family in assisting the child with cerebral palsy to lead a productive, satisfying life. *Children with cerebral palsy* includes contributions from doctors, therapists, educators, and parents, all of whom provide useful information and support. Information on many topics, including diagnosis, assessment, treatments, development, daily care, and legal rights is provided. The authors also deal with grief, anger and guilt in a compassionate and open manner. A glossary of important terms, reading list, and resource guide are included.

Hunt, Mimi, & Weiss, Sally (Eds.) *Each of us remembers... Parents of children with cerebral palsy answer your questions.* (32 pgs).

This booklet offers a chance for several parents to share with others what they've learned about having a child with cerebral palsy. Each parent answers questions that they wanted to ask when they received their children's diagnoses. Also included is a list of terms, with clear definitions, that are used in a diagnosis of cerebral palsy. The aim of this booklet is not only to answer questions, but to help new parents of children with cerebral palsy realize that they are not alone in the struggles that they face.

Down Syndrome

Pueschel, Siegfried M. (1990). *A parent's guide to Down's Syndrome: Toward a brighter future.* Baltimore, MD: Paul H. Brookes. (315 pgs).

>The author of this sensitive guide is the parent of a child with Down Syndrome. He has helped families around the world in coping with Down Syndrome. Pueschel discusses important developmental changes in the child and significant steps from infancy to adolescence. He provides simple explanations and advice on many pertinent topics. Sibling relationships, explanations to outsiders, educational considerations, and future quality of life are openly discussed with reassurance and strength. References and suggested readings are also included.

Stray-Gundersen, Karen (1986). *Babies with Down Syndrome.* Rockville, MD: Woodbine House. (235 pgs).

>Written by professionals and parents, this book covers everything new parents need to know about raising babies with Down Syndrome in a loving environment. Information on subjects important to the new parent, such as adjustment, daily care, and family life is explored with sensitivity and thoroughness. Also provided is a section on early intervention and the teaching of a baby with Down Syndrome.

Epilepsy

Reisner, Helen (1988). *Children with Epilepsy.* Rockville, MD: Woodbine House. (314 pgs).

>Vital current information and reassurance are offered in this volume to parents who face a long-misunderstood condition. The author gives a thorough explanation of epilepsy and discusses strategies for adjusting to this disorder. Important subjects such as development of high self-esteem in the epileptic child and the assessment of special needs are explored in a clear and compassionate style. A reading list, cassette list, and resource guide are also included.

General Topics

Anderson, Winifred, Chitwood, Stephan, & Hayden, Deidre (1990). *Negotiating the special education maze: A guide for parents and teachers.* Rockville, MD: Woodbine House. (269 pgs).

>This well-organized, step-by-step guide is a valuable tool for anyone who works with the special education system or is involved in the education of a child with special needs. The guide discusses strategies for helping parents to be effective advocates for their children. Suggestions are also given for ways they can participate in educational decisions that concern them. Included is a wide range of current information on special education services and options, as well as checklists, exercises, and charts. Each step in the special education process is explained clearly and thoroughly. Appendices include state and federal agencies and organizations dealing with specific disabilities.

*Batshaw, Mark L., & Perret, Yvonne M. (1993). *Children with disabilities: A medical primer.* Baltimore, MD: Paul H. Brookes. (664 pgs).

>This universal resource book offers vital information on causes and effects of disabling conditions, characteristics of specific disabilities, and diagnostic and intervention strategies. Also explored are contemporary societal issues affecting children and families. Illustrations, charts, graphs, case studies, a glossary, and a section on syndromes are included.

Bérard, Guy (1993). *Hearing equals behavior.* New Canaan, CT: Keats. (178 pgs).

>In this book, Dr. Bérard explains the auditory training approach he developed. This approach has been helpful to people who have conditions such as hyperactivity, dyslexia, suicidal depression, and autism. He discusses the nature of the hearing process, and several hearing disorders and their impact on behavior. He also explains how he developed and applied the auditory training approach, tells how to determine if an individual's behavior problems are caused by hearing problems, and discusses the apparatus used for testing and training. [Also see *The sound of a miracle* by Annabel Stehli, listed in the "Children with Special Needs" section.]

Callanan, Charles R. (1990). *Since Owen: A parent to parent guide for the care of the disabled child.* Baltimore, MD: Johns Hopkins Press. (466 pgs).

>Unique in its "family approach" to raising a child with disabilities, *Since Owen* gives parents informa-

tion they need. It answers a wide range of specific questions and suggests further resources that can help parents become knowledgeable partners with their child's professionals. It explores topics ranging from genetic counseling to placement in an institution and causes of birth defects to raising a child with special needs. A concluding section looks at the disabled child as an adult and discusses topics such as living arrangements and religion. Most importantly, it gives families the message that they are not alone.

Des Jardins, Charlotte (1993). *How to get services by being assertive.* Chicago, IL: Family Resource Center on Disabilities. (208 pgs).

This book, written for parents of children with disabilities and the professionals who work with them, offers helpful advice for all caregivers who need and/or desire services for a care receiver. Readers of this book will learn the difference between assertive and non-assertive behaviors; ways to develop positive attitudes and eliminate negative ones; and how to use assertiveness in working with professionals, bureaucrats and public officials. The author includes several success stories and information on available resources for parents and professionals.

Des Jardins, Charlotte (1993). *How to organize an effective parent/advocacy group and move bureaucracies.* Chicago, IL: Family Resource Center on Disabilities. (270 pgs).

Written for parents of children with disabilities and the professionals who work with them, this practical handbook is for any caregiver who wishes to become an advocate for caregivers and care receivers. The author offers helpful tips on how to set up parent/advocacy groups, effectively move bureaucracies to attain services, and teach children to become advocates for themselves by being positive and assertive. She also includes several success stories and helpful information on laws and legislation for parents, professionals, and children. A list of parent training and information centers and federal agencies is included.

Dickman, Irving R. (1993). *One miracle at a time: Getting help for a child with a disability* (rev. ed.). New York, NY: Fireside. (383 pgs).

This inspiring handbook offers the most recent information available on the new developments that are changing the future for disabled children, from saving at-risk newborns, to advances in assistive technology, to the pros and cons of full inclusion in education. This book not only provides practical advice and encouragement for parents of disabled children, but also includes an extensive resource list of support organizations and associations.

Fitton, Pat (1994). *Listen to me: Communicating the needs of people with profound intellectual and multiple disabilities.* Bristol, PA: Jessica Kingsley Publishers. (244 pgs).

Listen to me is a practical guide for parents and professionals coping with the complex problems of people with multiple disabilities. It offers information on asserting their rights, interpreting their needs successfully, and maintaining effective contact with professionals and organizations who deal with them. Pat Fitton uses examples from her own personal experiences with her disabled daughter to show how important it is to communicate that person's rights and needs in particular situations. She shows how it is possible to enrich the life of a person with profound disabilities and ensure that others value the person as an individual.

McAnaney, Kate Divine (1992). *I wish: Dreams and realities of parenting a special needs child.* Sacramento, CA: UCPA of California. (87 pgs).

This is a book about conflict, courage, and creative solutions. McAnaney tells what it's like to be the parent of a disabled child, and gives new perspective to professionals who work with exceptional families. In a conversational style, the author addresses guilt, grief, relaxation, and patience. Also included are messages from adults with disabilities who offer hope and inspiration.

McWilliam, P. J. (1993). *Working together with children and families.* Baltimore, MD: Paul H. Brookes. (310 pgs).

All of the case studies in this book are based on actual experiences of professionals working in early intervention with families of children with disabilities. Written in a narrative format, the case studies are more comparable to short stories than academic readings. The characteristics of the children and families are diverse, as are the settings in which services are provided. This book offers clear pictures of children without labels, families with unique values, and professionals with feelings of their own.

Rainforth, Beverly (1992). *Collaborative teams for students with severe disabilities.* Baltimore, MD: Paul H. Brookes. (284 pgs).

> Educational teams serving students with severe disabilities are entering an exciting and challenging era. Educational team members now have opportunities to play significant roles in assisting children and youths with severe disabilities to achieve fulfilling, integrated lives. The authors of this book discuss the philosophical, legal, and programmatic foundations of collaborative teamwork, the process of designing individualized education programs, and implementation strategies and issues.

Seligman, Milton (1989). *Ordinary families, special children.* New York: Guilford. (272 pgs).

> Families with children who have a disability are just like other families; however, the crisis of giving birth to a child with a disability thrusts family members into a situation that may make their lives different from those of other families. Discussions of this situation include social systems and family systems, becoming the parent of a disabled child, continuing adaptation, effects on family, models of intervention, cultural reactions, and professional-family interaction.

Simons, Robin (1987). *After the tears: Parents talk about raising a child with a disability.* San Diego, CA: Harcourt Brace Jovanovich. (89 pgs).

> In this book, Simons helps parents decide that they can continue to lead the lives they had planned—and incorporate their special needs children into it. Included are stories of parents who have chosen this path, sharing their experiences and offering encouragement. Subjects such as guilt and anger, sorrow, personal growth, marital stress, and the future are explored with sensitivity.

*Turnbull, Ann P., Patterson, Joan M., Behr, Shirley K., Murphy, Douglas L., Marquis, Janet G. & Blue-Banning, Martha J. (1993). *Cognitive coping, families, and disability.* Baltimore, MD: Paul H. Brookes. (321 pgs).

> *Cognitive coping, families, and disability* provides insights into family adjustment and adaptation to stress, research findings on coping strategies, and determinants of individual coping and coping style. Through a participatory research process, the authors gained valuable information on empirical, theoretical, clinical, and consumer perspectives about disability and cognitive coping. The book presents this information and provides professionals with a clear-cut research agenda.

Turnbull, Ann P., & Turnbull, III, H. Rutherford (1990). *Families, professionals, and exceptionality: A special partnership* (2nd ed.). New York: Merrill. (485 pgs).

> *Families, professionals, and exceptionality: A special partnership* concerns families, people who have disabilities, professionals, and ways they can work together more effectively. This book helps current and future professionals understand the diversity in families, family interaction, and family functions. Strategies for better communication between families and professionals are explored as well as ways to help families better cope with their situations. Professional ethics and morals are discussed, and when and if the use of the law is warranted. An extensive appendix with lists of resources for families and professionals is included.

Mental Retardation

Smith, Romayne (1993). *Children with mental retardation: A parent's guide.* Rockville, MD: Woodbine House. (437 pgs).

> This comprehensive guide covers mild to moderate retardation that has been diagnosed at birth or in early childhood. The authors discuss the emotional impact of the diagnosis on parents, as well as the challenges such a diagnosis presents. Thoroughly explored are subjects of development, evaluation, special education, and daily living of the mentally retarded child. Valuable strategies for coping and acceptance are presented for parents. Experiences of other families are expressed through parent statements to offer insight and reassurance to new parents of children with mental retardation.

Trainer, Marilyn (1991). *Differences in common: Straight talk on mental retardation, Down Syndrome, and life.* Rockville, MD: Woodbine House. (231 pgs)

> A collection of almost 50 essays, *Differences in common* speaks not only to a parent of a child that is

"different," but also to those who know little about people with mental retardation. Trainer brings a fresh, candid outlook to the challenges, hopes, and fears of family life—a life shaped by a child with Down Syndrome, but one which strikes a common chord in all of us.

Chronic Illness

*Biegel, David E., Sales, Esther, & Schulz, Richard (1991). *Family caregiving in chronic illness.* Newbury Park, CA: Sage. (331 pgs).

This volume provides a comprehensive analysis of the role and function of family caregiving within and across adult populations with dependency needs because of chronic disease. Five specific diseases are examined: cancer, heart disease, stroke, Alzheimer's disease, and mental illness. The authors provide a synthesis of existing research knowledge about family caregiving of dependent adult populations and suggest new directions for research and practice. Trends leading to the emergence of caregiving are carefully examined as a major societal issue. Intervention models are examined as well as research findings pertaining to the effectiveness of particular interventions.

Funk, Sandra G. (1993). *Key aspects of caring for the chronically ill.* New York: Springer. (350 pgs).

This comprehensive source book contains information on many aspects of caring for the chronically ill. In the overview, authors include discussions of hospitalized chronically ill, transitions from hospital to home, home care, living with chronic illness and research findings regarding the chronically ill. There is a special section covering issues concerning chronically ill children.

Goldfarb, Lori A., Brotherson, Mary Jane, Summers, Jean Ann, & Turnbull, Ann P. (1986). *Meeting the challenge of disability or chronic illness: A family guide.* Baltimore, MD: Paul H. Brookes. (181 pgs).

This practical tool for family problem solving can help ease the pain of difficult times and turn disappointments into triumphs. Part I, *Taking Stock*, will help families dealing with disability or chronic illness take an "inventory" of their family, identify their values and the resources available to them, and further strengthen those resources. Part II, *Problem Solving*, is a carefully thought-out process based on simplicity. The step-by-step method will help families to more quickly find solutions to the issues they face.

*Lyons, Renee F., Sullivan, Michael J. L., & Ritvo, Paul G. (1995). *Relationships in chronic illness and disability.* Thousand Oaks, CA: Sage. (189 pgs).

This book deals with the interpersonal issues that arise when relationships evolve under the challenges of chronic illness. Three interactive relationship-illness processes are examined: relationship change, supports and stressors, and relationship-focused coping. Also intervention in close relationships to improve coping with illness is discussed.

Maurer, Janet R. (1989). *Building a new dream.* New York, NY: Addison-Wesley Publishing Company. (307 pgs).

Building a new dream is a compassionate and practical guide to understanding and coping with the emotional and social aspects of chronic illness and disability. The author explains how to work with health professionals to learn about your illness and find resources, how to come to terms with emotional strain in order to cope with depression, and how to cope with the changing roles that illness brings about for all involved.

Pitzele, Sefra K. (1985). *We are not alone: Learning to live with chronic illness.* New York, NY: Workman. (315 pgs)

We are not alone offers inspiration and practical living strategies to millions of Americans suffering from chronic illnesses, and priceless advice for those who care for them. Drawing on firsthand experiences, the author is a friendly guide to coping with every aspect of chronic impairment, from overcoming the trauma of the diagnosis to managing daily routines with humor, dignity, and hope.

*Pollin, Irene, & Golant, Susan K. (1994). *Taking charge: Overcoming the challenges of long-term illness.* New York, NY: Random House. (255 pgs).

In *Taking charge*, the authors explain the method of Medical Crisis Counseling, which Ms. Pollin pioneered to help people survive the crisis of long-term illness and live productively. Eight common fears (fear of loss of control, fear of abandonment, fear of death, etc.) of those dealing with long-term illness are identified, and strategies are provided to help overcome them.

Register, Cheri (1987). *Living with chronic illness: Days of patience and passion.* New York, NY: Free Press. (316 pgs).

Living with chronic illness explores the shifting emotions involved in dealing with chronic illness, including the confusion and uncertainty that precede diagnosis and the unexpected relief that often comes when the nature of the illness is finally confirmed. Register illuminates patience as a way of life and discusses how it feels to know that disease will always be there. She also acknowledges that anger, fear, and grief can be appropriate, healthy responses to physical suffering.

Strong, Maggie (1988). *Mainstay: For the well spouse of the chronically ill.* New York, NY: Penguin Books. (329 pgs).

Mainstay is a book about living with a chronically ill spouse. Maggie Strong tells her own story and shows that living with someone who is chronically ill is more than just hard work. She raised her family, managed her house and family finances, maintained her career, and safeguarded her own emotional and physical needs while caring for her husband who has multiple sclerosis. Ms. Strong writes of the emotional toll experienced from keeping anger and guilt tucked away to being constantly aware that the situation will only get worse. The chapters are full of concrete, vital information on how to cope with the challenges of long-term illnesses. *Mainstay* is a book that will inspire courage and strength in all those who live with people who are chronically ill.

*Walsh, Froma, & Anderson, Carol M. (Eds.). (1988). *Chronic disorders and the family.* New York, NY: Haworth Press. (183 pgs).

The authors examine the role of the family in understanding and treating severe and chronic mental and physical illnesses. The goal is to increase awareness of the problems facing families coping with severe disorders. Topics such as schizophrenia, depression, anxiety disorders, eating disorders, and substance abuse are thoroughly explored, including research findings and therapy strategies.

Congregational Caregiving

Building Community Supports Project (1994). *Dimensions of faith and congregational ministries with persons with developmental disabilities and their families.* Piscataway, NJ: The University Affiliated Program of New Jersey. (56 pgs).

This guide includes a bibliography and a list of addresses of resources for clergy, laypersons, families, and service providers. These resources are divided by areas of interest and program/ministry. Examples of topics and information included are worship and sacraments, theological issues, parents and families of persons with disabilities, youth groups and adult education, pastoral counseling, and reading and audio/visual resources.

Harbaugh, Gary L. (1992). *Caring for the caregiver: Growth models for professional leaders and congregations.* Washington, DC: Alban Institute. (117 pgs).

This book is especially aimed at the clergy, reminding them of their responsibility to care for themselves as well as for others. It challenges congregations and churches to provide preventive care and ongoing support as well as crisis intervention. Helpful information at the end of the book includes a "caring for the caregiver" survey and a listing of resources.

Ransom, Judy G. (1994). *The courage to care: Seven families touched by disability and congregational caring.* Nashville, TN: Upper Room Books. (205 pgs).

This book is a collection of stories about seven different families who are struggling with different disabilities and finding help through congregational caring. Each story is unique and moving, but all demonstrate the impact of caring congregations during times of difficulty. Appendices include guidelines for helping and a listing of resources and organizations.

Coping and Self-Care for the Caregiver

Carter, Rosalynn (1994). *Helping yourself help others: A book for caregivers.* New York, NY: Times Books. (278 pgs).

Helping yourself help others was written to inform, encourage, empathize with, and advocate for informal (family and lay) caregivers. It also provides valuable insights for professional caregivers. Mrs. Carter discusses the feelings of caregivers; provides information about what caring means; explains the stages of caregiving; and offers ideas, information and advice to people currently providing care and to future caregivers. This guidebook offers practical solutions to caregivers' typical problems. It was written with empathy and sensitivity to help caregivers meet a difficult challenge head-on and find fulfillment and empowerment in their caregiving roles. Over 50 pages are devoted to addresses and phone numbers of organizations and a list of books helpful to caregivers.

Cole, Harry A. (1991). *Helpmates: Support in times of critical illness.* Louisville, KY: Westminster/John Knox Press. (157 pgs).

In this book, written by a caregiving spouse for other caregivers, author Harry Cole recognizes that caregivers who provide help for dependent loved ones are often unprepared to cope with the physical and emotional effects that accompany long-term illness. Making use of interviews with many people involved in caring for loved ones who are critically or terminally ill, Cole gives direction and support to help caregivers gain more patience and understanding.

Collins, Sheila K. (1992). *Stillpoint: The dance of self-caring, self-healing.* Fort Worth, TX: TLC Productions. (201 pgs).

Stillpoint is a practical self-help book for anyone who is a caregiver at work and/or in family life. The author states that people who care for others often have trouble caring for themselves (physically, mentally, emotionally and spiritually) and that failure to care for oneself may lead to loss of ability to care for others. The book will help readers increase their understanding of themselves; identify the missing elements in their self-caring lifestyles; learn how to alter their environments to support self-care; and learn self-caring skills to take care of themselves while caring for others.

Dempcy, Mary, & Tihista, Rene (1991). *Stress personalities: A look inside our selves.* Bolinas, CA: Focal Point Press. (233 pgs).

This book discusses seven types of stress personalities many people possess, and their effects on relationships and health. The book helps readers identify their own stress personalities and learn how these affect their lives. At the end of each section, the authors offer new, positive behaviors to practice in order to counteract the respective stress personality behaviors which are unproductive and detrimental.

Hover, Margot (1994). *Caring for yourself when caring for others.* Mystic, CT: Twenty-Third Publications. (74 pgs).

The author uses scripture, personal stories, situational experiences and prayer to offer practical and uplifting support for caregivers. She offers simple, direct advice for dealing with everyday occurrences facing those who give care to others. She also offers ways that caregivers can nourish themselves and revitalize their efforts.

Karr, Katherine L. (1992). *Taking time for me: How caregivers can effectively deal with stress.* Buffalo, NY: Prometheus Books. (175 pgs).

Family caregivers must often juggle their duties as parents, spouses, and employees while tending to the daily needs of a loved one who is elderly, chronically ill, or dying. For these people, stress often becomes an everyday occurrence that at times seems insurmountable. Karr's insightful observations and suggestions—enhanced by personal accounts of real care providers who are struggling with their own needs while tending to the needs of others—demonstrate that caregivers can overcome their personal conflicts and develop innovative ways of renewing their strength without jeopardizing the well-being of those who depend on them.

Kleinke, Chris L. (1990). *Coping with life challenges.* Pacific Grove, CA: Brooks/Cole. (240 pgs).

This easy-to-understand guide helps the reader learn to cope with illness, pain, loss, anger, failure, and conflict. Whether the difficulties are minor or serious, presented in this book are coping strategies that can help anyone regain a sense of control in his or her life. The author presents a "how-to" approach and practical suggestions for making the information work for the reader.

Schafer, Walt (1992). *Stress management for wellness* (2nd ed.). Orlando, FL: Harcourt. (533 pgs).

This book will prove helpful for every person, but especially to caregivers who are experiencing significant stress in their lives. It promotes an integrated, whole person, lifestyle approach to stress management. Its goal is to assist readers to control and channel stress rather than succumb to it. Aspects of stress and coping included in this book are: understanding stress and wellness, stress related symptoms and disorders, Type A behavior and hostility, and methods of managing stress. Special applications applying to college stress and job stress are also included. Many tables, self-rating scales and self-help exercises help readers analyze their own stress and coping behaviors.

Schlossberg, Nancy K. (1994). *Overwhelmed: Coping with life's ups and downs.* New York, NY: Lexington. (154 pgs).

All of us face transitions or turning points in our lives. How we handle these journeys, live through them, and learn from them is what this book is about. The author discusses the transition process, how to take stock of your situation and yourself, and how to take charge of the changes in your life. Her prescription for coping is mature, sympathetic, and realistic.

Sherman, James R. (1994). *Creative caregiving.* Golden Valley, MN: Pathway Books (84 pgs).

This book helps caregivers to develop creative ways to relieve the difficult aspects of their caregiving. The author discusses: creativity and caregiving, barriers to creative caregiving, the seven components needed for creativity, and how to develop your creative talents. Check lists and exercises help the reader become a more creative caregiver.

Sherman, James R. (1995). *The magic of humor in caregiving.* Golden Valley, MN: Pathway Books. (93 pgs).

This book explains the well-established healing benefits of laughter and humor in reducing stress. It shows how playfulness and humor can be used to increase personal effectiveness, promote wellness and lighten the impact of one's caregiving. Self-rating check lists and self-help exercises help readers evaluate the extent to which humor is currently a part of their lives and helps them learn how to increase the laughter in their lives.

Sherman, James R. (1994). *Positive caregiver attitudes.* Golden Valley, MN: Pathway Books. (84 pgs).

This is an important manual for any caregiver. It is loaded with down-to-earth strategies for developing and maintaining positive attitudes toward care receivers, caregiving and life in general. This book also identifies the sources of negative feelings and illustrates their destructive effects. It is filled with simple rules, common sense ideas, and self-help exercises.

Sherman, James R. (1994). *Preventing caregiver burnout.* Golden Valley, MN: Pathway Books. (76 pgs).

Caregivers work long hours under constant emotional pressure and can lose their motivation and commitment to caregiving. This book addresses this fact. It describes what burnout is, what causes it, and the effects it has on the burned-out person. Lastly, the author presents easy-to-follow procedures for preventing burnout and maintaining an optimistic outlook toward caregiving. Check lists and self-help exercises are included.

Spencer, Sabina A., & Adams, John D. (1990). *Life changes: Growing through personal transitions.* San Luis Obispo, CA: Impact. (192 pgs).

Helping readers cope with the inevitable personal transitions in life is the focus of this book. Caregivers can use *Life changes* as a tool to give them suggestions for coping with their caregiving demands. The contents include: life changes, the seven stages of transition, where to find support, developing and utilizing skills to deal with change, keeping a positive attitude, staying healthy, managing stress, and living with change.

Diabetes

*Krall, Leo P. (1989). *Joslin diabetes manual.* Malvern, PA: Lea & Febiges. (406 pgs).

This instructional guide is full of detailed information concerning people with diabetes. Its aim is to assist diabetics to understand the disorder, and to learn how to live full and healthy lives. The author thoroughly describes the process of diabetes, the different types, and their causes and symptoms. The issues of nutrition, exercise, treatments, and pregnancy are also covered in the chapters.

Eating Disorders

*Brownell, Kelly D., & Foreyt, John P. (Eds.). (1986). *Handbook of eating disorders: Physiology, psychology and treatment of obesity, anorexia, and bulimia.* New York, NY: BasicBooks. (529 pgs).

This book is an important resource for professionals who work with people who have eating disorders—anorexia, bulimia, and obesity. Written by authorities in the field, it focuses on all aspects of these disorders—health consequences, epidemiology, inpatient and outpatient treatment.

Siegel, Michele, Brisman, Judith, & Weinshel, Margot (1988). *Surviving an eating disorder: Strategies for family and friends.* New York, NY: Harper & Row. (222 pgs).

This book offers specific guidelines to help family and friends of people who have eating disorders. The authors offer rules and new behaviors/actions which will encourage the recovery process. Psychological components of eating disorders and possible treatments are discussed. Other helpful books and organizations are included. Topics of this book include: the behavioral, psychological and family context of eating disorders; bringing the disorder out in the open; coping with denial; seeking help; disengaging from the eating disorder; and relating to the person, not the disorder.

Elderly as Caregivers

*Minkler, Meredith (1993). *Grandmothers as caregivers.* Newbury Park, CA: Sage. (238 pgs).

This book contains discussions exploring the concerns of grandmothers as caregivers. The author looks at the health status of grandmother caregivers, economic considerations, support networks and social support, combining work and child care, raising children of the crack cocaine epidemic, and community interventions to support grandparent caregivers.

*Roberto, Karen A. (Ed.). (1993). *The elderly caregiver: Caring for adults with developmental disabilities.* Newbury Park, CA: Sage. (216 pgs).

Roberto addresses the predominant issues and concerns confronting elder caregivers. She provides insight into the physical, psychological, and social needs of this growing segment of the population. The needs of elderly people caring for adult children, aging adults, and persons with specific disabilities are explored including the increasing burden of caregiving, the ordeal of facing their own future, and planning for out-of-home placement. Case management is also examined.

General Topics

Bass, Deborah S. (1990). *Caring families: Supports and interventions.* Washington, DC: National Association of Social Workers. (279 pgs).

In this volume, Bass provides a useful framework for understanding and assisting those who care for family members—both young and old. This book provides useful practice tools for assessing the strengths and needs of caregiving families, and for assisting them in problem solving and in coping with the stresses of caregiving. *Caring families* will be important to many audiences: helping professionals, public and private policymakers, and caregiving families. Addresses and phone numbers of state agencies such as Medicaid, aging, maternal and child health, developmental disabilities, special education; VA medical centers and clinics; and Department of Defense family support programs are included.

*Boise, Linda (Ed.). (No date). *Helping families help themselves: Reaching the employed caregiver.* Portland, OR: Family Support Services, Good Samaritan Hospital & Medical Center. (15 pgs).

This booklet is for people and organizations that provide support or are considering developing programs for employed caregivers, or who would like to know more about the special needs of working caregivers. It identifies their needs, offers information about programs and services which can help them, and offers advice on ways to reach them through the workplace and community programs. Topics include: a profile of the employed caregiver, the challenges of working and caregiving, what employed caregivers need, benefits to business, how a survey can assess need, how focus groups help, ways to reach employed caregivers, offering programs in the workplace, and sample telephone scripts, letters, questions, and evaluation forms.

Caplan, Paula J. (1994). *You're smarter than they make you feel: How the experts intimidate us and what we can do about it.* New York, NY: Free Press. (212 pgs).

> Drawing on a wealth of anecdotes along with current psychological research, Paula Caplan persuasively shows us that we do not need to feel stupid or powerless when dealing with experts in any field. She points out the techniques experts typically use to intimidate clients, why they employ these techniques, and why we blame ourselves. Caplan concludes by showing us how we can recognize the techniques of disempowerment, employ helpful counter strategies, and think more critically in order to elicit the needed information or action.

*Cicirelli, Victor G. (1992). *Family caregiving: Autonomous and paternalistic decision making.* Newbury Park, CA: Sage. (252 pgs).

> *Family caregiving* offers researchers, practitioners, and professionals an informative look at a new area of inquiry—paternalism and respect for autonomy in family caregiving decision making. It clearly discusses family caregiving in long-term home care, the meaning of autonomy and paternalism, and the nature of dyadic family decision making. This volume emphasizes autonomy in family care as opposed to formal care and how lack of education, negative attitudes towards elders, and family traditions can influence the frequency of paternalistic decision making.

Committee on Handicaps (1993). *Caring for people with physical impairment: The journey back.* Washington, DC: American Psychiatric Press. (178 pgs).

> This book brings together the expertise of caregivers from a variety of backgrounds to examine the special needs of patients with physical impairments. It explores clinical and educational applications to the caregiving of the physically impaired. Offered in this volume is information on coping strategies for the caregiver and on the special issues related to the rehabilitation process. The information will be helpful to both informal and formal caregivers.

Doka, K. J. (1993). *Living with life-threatening illness: A guide for patients, their families, and caregivers.* New York, NY: Lexington Books.

> Provided in this book is a positive plan for improving the lives of seriously ill patients, their families, and caregivers. *Living with life-threatening illness* gives us a new way of looking at the different stages of illness. The experience of living with illness is emphasized, rather than just anticipating its terminal phase. This book is essential for all who are dealing with major illness, whether personally or professionally.

*Feetham, Suzanne L., Meister, Susan B., Bell, Janice M., & Gilliss, Catherine L. (Eds.). (1993). *The nursing of families: Theory/research/education/practice.* Newbury Park, CA: Sage. (308 pgs).

> *The nursing of families* offers significant directions for cross-cutting issues in practice, education, research and theory to help bridge the gap between perceived needs and expectations of families, and the actual practice of nursing. Among the issues explored are policy and economic issues, theory development, research methodology, cross-cultural concerns, HIV/AIDS, and homeless mothers and children.

*Gaut, Delores A. (1992). *The presence of caring in nursing.* Hudson Street, NY: National League for Nursing Press. (267 pgs).

> This book is a collection of essays dealing with the topic of caring in nursing. Explored are the concepts of presence, spiritual connection, caring nursing environments, impact of nurses' caring on patients, conflict between caring and professionalization, and the magic of caring.

Gething, Lindsay (1992). *Person to person: A guide for professionals working with people with disabilities.* Baltimore, MD: Paul H. Brookes.

> Gething looks at a great many aspects of different types of disabilities: physiology; treatment; social and emotional aspects; family reactions; education; employment; attitudes of others; and much more. Written with personal accounts, this guide is easy to read and sympathetic. It would be useful for the professional or the layperson who would like to learn more about the different aspects of impairment.

Grasha, Anthony F. (1995). *Practical applications of psychology* (4th ed.). New York, NY: HarperCollins. (476 pgs).

> This book explores how psychology may be applied to the individual in everyday life. Readers are shown how to develop action plans to help them make

more effective decisions, modify their behavior, communicate and relate to others better, manage stress, and develop positive self-images. Family caregivers would also find this text helpful.

*Hayslip, Bert (1992). *Hospice care.* Newbury Park, CA: Sage. (235 pgs).

The intent of this volume is to serve as an introduction to hospice for new personnel, students, and volunteers. Its focus is toward the nonmedical aspects of patient care. Addressed are the issues of communication and assessment skills in hospice, special education role of hospice, working with the patient, working with families, and grief and bereavement.

Heath, Angela (1993). *Long distance caregiving: A survival guide for far away caregivers.* Lakewood, CO: American Source Books. (122 pgs).

Long distance caregiving is a helpful guide which provides step-by-step, practical suggestions for caregivers, especially caregivers who live some distance from their care receivers. Some of the topics included are: travel tips, paperwork, legal and financial issues, adjusting your care plan, and relocation. Check lists of suggestions, tips and considerations, and what should be done within specific time frames help organize caregivers. A list of helpful organizations appears at the end.

*Hooyman, Nancy R., & Gonyea, Judith (1995). *Feminist perspectives on family care: Policies for gender justice.* Thousand Oaks, CA: Sage. (418 pgs).

In *Feminist perspectives on family care*, the authors examine caregiving as a feminist issue, looking at its impact on women socially, personally, and economically. They review how changing family structures, the changing economy and workforce, and the changing health care demands of needy adults have affected women's lives. They also critique existing public and private policies, and the changes in social institutions and attitudes meant to improve the lives of women.

Horowitz, Karen E., & Lanes, Douglas M. (1992). *Witness to illness: Strategies for caregiving and coping.* Reading, MA: Addison-Wesley. (277 pgs).

Witness to illness speaks to our feelings of helplessness, and perhaps hopelessness, when we are unable to do anything to restore health to a loved one. Horowitz and Lanes show us that we don't have to be passive. This book follows the course of events in a typical illness—from handling the initial bad news, through caregiving, to the long-term effects of the illness—and suggests specific, practical ways in which we can actively contribute to the survival and well-being of people we care for and about.

*Kahana, Eva, Biegel, David E., & Wykle, May L. (1994). *Family caregiving across the lifespan.* Thousand Oaks, CA: Sage. (418 pgs).

Family caregiving across the lifespan considers the broad spectrum of chronic illnesses that require family caregiving throughout the lifespan and includes in its focus both members of the family caregiving relationship and significant non-family caregivers. The authors also explore the social context in which care is provided, devoting an entire section to discussions of interaction between informal and formal caregivers and society at large. The value of providing support to caregivers, including caregivers of persons with AIDS, is discussed.

Larson, Dale G. (1993). *The helper's journey: Working with people facing grief, loss, and life threatening illness.* Champaign, IL: Research Press. (279 pgs).

This book is for caregivers—professional and family. It is divided into three main sections. Part 1 focuses on the personal experiences of helping, such as emotional involvement and handling stress. Part 2 discusses the interpersonal dimensions of caregiving, focusing on helping relationships and communication skills. Part 3 deals with helping teams and support groups and how they can benefit healing.

*Lassiter, Sybil M. (1995). *Multicultural clients: A professional handbook for health care providers and social workers.* Westport, CT: Greenwood Press. (194 pgs).

This text provides basic information to health care providers who work with multicultural clients. The author presents the following cultural groups: African, Arab, Chinese, Cuban, East Indian, Filipino, German, Haitian, Irish, Italian, Japanese, Jewish, Korean, Mexican, and Vietnamese Americans and discusses their population numbers, economic status, major illnesses and death rates in the USA. Lassiter makes comparisons of orientations toward family, the elderly, child rearing, socialization, health beliefs and practices, dietary patterns, religious beliefs and practices, and beliefs about death and dying for each cultural group.

*Lechner, Viola M., & Creedon, Michael A. (1994). *Managing work and family life.* New York, NY: Springer. (187 pgs).

In this addition to the professional literature on the changing needs of families and working caregivers, the authors identify and discuss emerging family-sensitive corporate- and government-sponsored programs and employee benefits. They describe the full range of workplace responses and focus on policies (e.g., the Family Medical Leave Act of 1993) and programs (e.g., flextime, job sharing, and compressed work weeks). Lechner and Creedon delineate a seven-step program-development model for labor unions and companies interested in planning and implementing family-focused workplace programs.

*Locke, Don C. (1992). *Increasing multicultural understanding: A comprehensive model.* Newbury Park, CA: Sage. (166 pgs).

This book sets forth the process necessary to implement effective education and counseling strategies for culturally diverse populations. It is designed to provide one of the necessary steps in accomplishing the task of gaining an overview of various cultural groups. It will help the reader identify characteristics of cultures, make comparisons between the dominant culture and culturally different groups, and use that information to develop strategies or interventions for students or clients. Readers will become more aware of their own ethnocentrism and increase their awareness of the role culture plays in determining the ways people think, feel, and act.

Lowe, Paula C. (1993). *Carepooling: How to get the help you need to care for the ones you love.* San Francisco, CA: Berrett-Koehler Publishers. (292 pgs).

Carepooling offers simple, practical ways to exchange help and share support with friends, neighbors and co-workers. Enlivened by stories of over 200 caregivers, this book provides the tools to: identify potential carepoolers, understand why it's hard to ask for help, initiate carepooling relationships, resolve conflicts among carepoolers, and hire a shared care provider.

Lustbader, Wendy (1991). *Counting on kindness: The dilemmas of dependency.* New York, NY: The Free Press. (206 pgs).

Vividly illustrated with true stories and quotations, and full of insights from Wendy Lustbader's clinical experience, *Counting on Kindness* explores issues of power and dependency and shows how to regain a sense of power and purpose while dependent on others. She discusses such issues as coping with too much time on one's hands, learning to think of the past productively, handling regret and feelings of uselessness, and reviving one's self esteem in the face of dependency.

*MacNamara, Roger Dale (1992). *Creating abuse-free caregiving environments for children, the disabled, and the elderly: Preparing, supervising, and managing caregivers for the emotional impact of their responsibilities.* Springfield, IL: Charles C. Thomas. (256 pgs).

MacNamara takes the position that professional caregivers must be able, stable and self-renewing to avoid becoming abusive. In this manual, the author explores the topic of abuse, its relationship to environment and stress, and describes a series of abuser "profiles." He also offers strategies for avoiding or stopping abusive behaviors.

Mayeroff, Milton (1990). *On caring.* New York, NY: Harper Collins. (123 pgs).

A generalized description of caring and an account of how caring can give comprehensive meaning and order to one's life are the themes dealt with in this book. It is a short, beautifully written account of what it means to live a full, happy and connected life and how to help others come to do this. Mayeroff makes the reader aware of what caring involves in a clear and engaging style.

McDaniel, Susan H., Hepworth, Jeri, & Doherty, William J. (1992). *Medical family therapy: A biopsychosocial approach to families with health problems.* New York, NY: BasicBooks. (295 pgs).

In *Medical family therapy*, the authors detail their medical family therapy model, a biopsychosocial family systems approach that operates in collaboration with patients, families, health care professionals and community groups. The goal is to coordinate care for the benefit of people who are ill and their families/caregivers.

*Maguire, Lambert (1991). *Social support systems in practice: A generalist approach.* Silver Spring, MD: National Association of Social Workers Press. (177 pgs).

> This book for social work practitioners is designed to be a practical guide to using social support systems. The author examines the variety of ways in which social work practitioners can organize family, friends, and fellow professionals into therapeutic, rehabilitative, or preventive units of help for clients. The book describes three different approaches to such social support systems but maintains a generalist orientation.

Miller, James E. (1995). *When you're the caregiver: 12 things to do if someone you care for is ill or incapacitated. When you're ill or incapacitated: 12 things to remember in times of sickness, injury or disability.* Ft. Wayne, IN: Willowgreen. (62 pgs).

> This book is written for the caregiver AND the care receiver. The author combines his knowledge as an ordained clergyman and grief counselor to help offer words of spiritual comfort and advice to help facilitate a cooperative, working partnership between the caregiver and care receiver and to increase each partner's ability to cope with the situation.

*Nisbet, Jan (1992). *Natural supports in school, at work, and in the community for people with severe disabilities.* Baltimore, MD: Paul H. Brookes. (362 pgs).

> Promoting the positions that assistance must be defined by the needs of individuals rather than the requirements of service "systems", this definitive book combines thoughtful research and provocative first-person accounts to give fresh insight and practical guidance for using natural supports. Thoughtful chapters supply essential information on strategies for building community membership for individuals with disabilities, on support programs and networks available, on the role of natural supports in public schools, and much more.

*Nottingham, Jack, & Nottingham, Joanne (Eds.). (1990). *The professional and family caregiver—Dilemmas, rewards, and new directions.* Americus, GA: Rosalynn Carter Institute for Human Development, Georgia Southwestern College. (77 pgs).

> The presentations given at the inaugural conference of the Rosalynn Carter Institute for Human Development in 1990 at Georgia Southwestern College in Americus, GA are contained in this book. Topics include: caregiving in America, shared responsibility, caring for the caregiver, caregiving in a holistic context, senior citizen caregivers, caring for the chronically and mentally ill, professional and family caregiving from medical and social work perspectives, health and mental health care in the future, and the caring community.

*Pugach, Marleen C., & Johnson, Lawrence J. (1995). *Collaborative practitioners/collaborative schools.* Denver, CO: Love Publishing. (265 pgs).

> This book stresses collaboration among professionals, families and students in schools. However, many of the principles are applicable to health care, its providers, caregiving families, and care receivers. The emphasis is on teamwork to enhance services and benefit the people involved. Topics include: collaboration (what it is, how to do it, and participation); communication (skills to facilitate, and barriers to, effective communication); and collaboration (working with and supporting groups, and school-university and school-family collaboration).

*Rolland, John S. (1994). *Families, illness and disability: An integrative treatment model.* New York, NY: BasicBooks. (309 pgs).

> Using his Family Systems Illness Model, the author shows how the biopsychosocial demands of different illnesses and disabilities create particular strains on the family, how the stages of an illness affect the family, how family legacies of loss and illness shape their coping responses, and how family belief systems play a crucial role in the ability to manage health and illness. Practitioners will learn how to help families: live well despite physical limitations and the uncertainties of threatened loss; encourage empowering rather than shame-based illness narratives; rewrite rigid caregiving scripts; and encourage intimacy and maximize autonomy for all family members. This is an ideal book for all health and mental health professionals and students who work with illness, disability, and loss in a wide variety of clinical settings.

Roter, Debra L., & Hall, Judith A. (1993). *Doctors talking with patients/patients talking with doctors: Improving communication in medical visits.* Westport, CT: Auburn House. (203 pgs).

> Medical visits are not as effective and satisfying as they would be if doctors and patients communicated better with each other. Roter and Hall set out specific, scientifically established principles and recommendations for improving doctor-patient relationships. Improved communication will aid understanding, improve motivation, encourage the pursuit of medical advice, and reduce negative psychological/emotional reactions, especially for patients.

*Salisbury, Christine L., & Intagliata, James (1986). *Respite care: Support for persons with developmental disabilities and their families.* Baltimore, MD: Paul H. Brookes. (315 pgs).

> This book is about providing respite care for families who have a member with a disability. *Respite care* represents an effort to respond to the growing need for information on respite care and family support services by providing readers with a perspective on the rationale for and design and evaluation of respite care programs. The chapters provide a wealth of practical information presented against a background of theory and research supporting the need for respite services. The reader will gain an understanding of the issues surrounding the establishment of respite programs.

*Sawa, Russell J. (Ed.). (1992). *Family health care.* Newbury Park, CA: Sage. (297 pgs).

> This collection presents an assortment of ways of talking about families, analyzing their effects on health and illness, and assessing the family coping strategies and how effective they are. In doing this, the author relates family pathology and therapy to concerns of primary care. Sections cover family theories and primary health care, research on family health care, and education and practice of professionals dealing with families.

*Schaufeli, Wilmar B., Maslach, Christina, & Marek, Tadeusz (Eds.). (1993). *Professional burnout: Recent developments in theory and research.* Washington, DC: Taylor & Francis. (292 pgs).

> A rapidly growing number of people experience psychological strain at their workplaces. Results of this include higher rates of absenteeism and turnover, and an increasing number of workers receiving disability benefits due to psychological problems. This book focuses on one specific kind of occupational stress: burnout, the depletion of energy resources as a result of continuous emotional demands of the job. There are five sections to the book: interpersonal approaches, individual approaches, organizational approaches, methodological issues, and the future outlook of burnout.

Shields, Craig V. (1987). *Strategies: A practical guide for dealing with professionals and human service systems.* Richmond Hill, Ontario: Human Services Press. (144 pgs).

> This handbook answers many common questions, discusses situations and problems typically faced when dealing with human service providers, and offers strategies for dealing with them. Shields helps the reader understand professionals and become familiar with the "system." Considerations for selecting a professional or agency and dealing with personnel are explored in detail. A particularly helpful master list of strategies is included in the appendix.

*Singer, George H.S., & Irvin, Larry K. (Eds.). (1989). *Support for caregiving families: Enabling positive adaptation to disability.* Baltimore, MD: Paul H. Brookes. (348 pgs).

> These authors present an overview of family support services for families of individuals with developmental disabilities. The services described in the book aim to create productive partnerships between social services and families in order to help families succeed in their caregiving roles without supplanting them. Content is organized around the roles of family stress and the concept of the family life cycle.

*Singer, George H. S., Powers, Laurie E., & Olson, Ardis L. (1996). *Redefining family support: Innovations in public-private partnerships.* Baltimore, MD: Paul H. Brookes. (477 pgs).

> This resource examines family support practices, policies, and strategies. It outlines various programs and funding options for meeting the diverse needs of families who care for a family member who has a disability. Topics include: family support for families of people with special needs, family support across populations, and issues and innovations in public policy.

*Stevenson, Robert G. (Ed.). (1994). *What will we do? Preparing a school community to cope with crises.* Amityville, NY: Baywood Publishing. (214 pgs).

> *What will we do?* was written to train school personnel to help victims cope with crises. Although this book is aimed at schools, health care and other professionals could benefit from the information, resources and techniques discussed. Topics include: preparing schools for crisis management; crises of youth suicide, HIV/AIDS, and violence; support groups and the role of peer support; and critical incident stress debriefing.

*Unger, Donald G., & Powell, Douglas R. (Eds.). (1991). *Families as nurturing systems: Support across the life span.* Binghamton, NY: Haworth. (251 pgs).

> In this volume, Unger and Powell recognize the power of the family when they characterize families as nurturing systems. This book deals with family support across the life span and within different settings. It prescribes new and more collaborative-oriented ways for practitioners to work with families. The purpose of the book is to refine and extend existing knowledge about approaches to supporting the caregiving roles of families across the life span.

*Wasik, Barbara Hanna (1990). *Home visiting.* Newbury Park, CA: Sage. (304 pgs)

> *Home visiting* represents one of the first modern attempts to present comprehensive information about procedures and issues related to home visiting with families. The author includes chapters on home visiting programs, personnel issues in home visiting, helping skills and techniques, visiting families in stressful situations, professional issues for home visitors, and future directions in home visiting.

*Zarit, Steven H., Pearlin, Leonard I., & Schaie, K. Warner (Eds.). (1993). *Caregiving systems: Formal and informal helpers.* Hillsdale, NJ: Lawrence Erlbaum Associates. (332 pgs).

> The authors address the topic of informal systems of care from a cultural perspective, considering the complexity of cultural contexts and their effect on care. The section on formal systems of care focuses on Social Health Maintenance Organizations and related public policy, home care services, barriers to use of services, and other related issues.

Loss and Grief

Bozarth, Alla R. (1990). *A journey through grief.* Center City, MN: Hazelden. (51 pgs).

> In the long and anguishing journey of grief after the loss of a loved one, Dr. Alla R. Bozarth sensitively brings a message of assurance, comfort, and hope. Dr. Bozarth will tell you what to expect, what to do, and what to think. She will help you understand the physical symptoms of grieving, and to express what the loss really means to you.

Bozarth, Alla R. (1986). *Life is goodbye, life is hello: Grieving well through all kinds of loss.* Minneapolis, MN: Compcare. (203 pgs).

> This author has guided others through all kinds of loss and disappointment: Separation and change; physical death; death of a relationship and even the death of a dream. Bozarth shows how to make grieving an action, and helps readers become agents in their own healing process rather than victims of their grief.

Doka, Kenneth J. (Ed.). (1995). *Children mourning, mourning children.* Washington, DC: Hospice Foundation of America. (179 pgs).

> This compassionate guide addresses the sensitive topic of children and grief. Death, life-threatening illness and mourning are discussed from a child's perspective. Strategies for answering children's questions and talking to children about illness are included. The final section explains research in the field of children and grief and provides information about literature for children on death, dying, and bereavement.

Doka, Kenneth J. (Ed.). (1996). *Living with grief after sudden loss.* Washington, DC: Hospice Foundation of America. (271 pgs).

> This book is the outgrowth of the 1996 teleconference, *Living with grief after sudden loss,* sponsored by the Hospice Foundation of America. The articles contained in this text will help professional caregivers give aid to families dealing with loss, grief and death. (It will also be beneficial to family members who have experienced the death of a loved one.) This book is specifically aimed at sudden loss, but anyone experiencing bereavement from any type of loss would be helped by some of the articles.

Kennedy, Alexandra (1991). *Losing a parent: Passage to a new way of living.* San Francisco, CA: Harper. (139 pgs).

> *Losing a parent* offers readers an array of suggestions and techniques that will enable them to deal more effectively with the grief that a loved one's death causes. The author guides readers through this intense life change, providing help for gaining insight and maintaining inner peace.

Lewis, C.S. (1961). *A grief observed.* New York, NY: HarperCollins. (80 pgs).

> *A grief observed* is a compilation of short journal-like entries which were written by a man mourning the loss of his wife. Writing this small book became "a defense against total collapse, a safety valve" and the author came to realize that "bereavement is a universal and integral part of our experience of love." This volume will help anyone who is dealing with grief and loss.

Livingston, Gordon (1995). *Only spring: On mourning the death of my son.* New York, NY: HarperCollins. (230 pgs).

> This journal was written by a father during the time his son was ill and dying and also after his death. It reveals the grief, helplessness, torment, hope, love, anguish and strain the family experienced while coping with his illness and death. This is a book of survival of those who live on. It offers suggestions about how to grieve, gain strength, and confront great and difficult challenges in life.

*Rando, Therese A. (1984). *Grief, dying and death.* Champaign, IL: Research Press Company. (476 pgs).

> Early chapters of this book address the issues of bereavement, attitudes toward loss, reactions to loss, and unresolved grief, why these things occur, and how to work with individuals and families who are hurting from a loss. The latter half of the book looks at the issues of terminal illness care. Dr. Rando presents a sensitive but realistic approach to the difficult issues to be faced in the dying process. She offers many practical suggestions for the caregiver who is working with both individuals and families.

Rando, Therese A. (1986). *Parental loss of a child.* Champaign, IL: Research Press Company. (555 pgs).

> Parental loss of a child is unlike any other loss. The grief of parents is particularly severe, complicated, and long-lasting, with major and unparalleled symptom fluctuations over time. Readable and insightful chapters discuss perspectives on the parental loss of a child, issues in specific types of death, socially unacknowledged parental bereavements, subjective experiences of death, professional help for bereaved parents, and organizations that can help.

*Todd, Andrew (Ed.). (1995). *Journey of the heart: Stories of grief as told by nurses in the NICU* (2nd ed.). Nashville, TN: Vanderbilt University Medical Center. (271 pgs).

> This book has two distinct parts. Part 1, which is emotional and moving, relates the stories nurses tell about their work, experiences, knowledge, emotions and insights as nurses in the Newborn Intensive Care Unit. Part 2 (Appendices) includes several helpful tools: a glossary, grief support and what is done for families, bereavement checklist and follow up, what to say and not to say to families in their time of grief, and resources and organizations.

Mental Illness

Depression

Berger, Diane, & Berger, Lisa (1991). *We heard the angels of madness: A family guide to coping with manic depression.* New York, NY: Quill, William, Morrow. (308 pgs).

> Diane and Lisa Berger share both the intimate and inspiring story of how their family coped with Mark's manic depressive illness and the valuable information they gathered about manic depression over the course of his treatment. Up-to-date facts on drugs, doctors, therapy, insurance and other resources are included. The authors discuss how to identify the symptoms of manic depression and avoid a false diagnosis, which treatments work and which don't, and the emotional experience of a mother battling for the sanity and well-being of her child.

Kerns, Lawrence L. (1993). *Helping your depressed child: A reassuring guide to the causes and treatments of childhood and adolescent depression.* Rocklin, CA: Prima Publishing. (284 pgs).

> Dr. Kerns explains why children get depressed and outlines the role that a parent or teacher can play in

helping a child deal constructively with these feelings. Also discussed are possible treatments for childhood depression—therapy, drug therapy, and hospitalization.

Klein, Donald F., & Wender, Paul H. (1993). *Understanding depression: A complete guide to its diagnosis and treatment.* New York, NY: Oxford University Press. (181 pgs).

>The authors offer a definitive guide to depressive illness—its causes, course and symptoms. They clarify the difference between depression (which is a normal emotion) and biological depression (which is an illness), and include several self-rating tests which readers can use to help determine whether or not they should seek psychiatric evaluation to establish if they have a biological depressive illness. Klein and Wender describe the symptoms of biological depression, how depressive illness can affect people's lives, and different types of treatment available.

General Topics

Esser, Aristide H., & Lacey, Sylvia D. (1989). *Mental illness: A homecare guide.* New York, NY: John Wiley & Sons. (263 pgs).

>This book was written to increase awareness of homecare alternatives in psychiatric treatment of chronic emotional and mental problems. It serves as a guide to help families reach homecare treatment decisions more decisively and comprehensively while remaining flexible in exploring various kinds of therapies and community support services. The authors show families what criteria to use in selecting professional services, and how to help design a treatment program, cope with unforeseen circumstances, ensure self-preservation, and assist their disturbed relatives or friends in living a productive and rewarding life. Practical and understandable step-by-step instructions are given for dealing with the day-to-day problems in the medical treatment and psychosocial education of the ill family member.

*Hatfield, Agnes B. (1990). *Family education in mental illness.* New York: Guilford. (211 pgs).

>This book provides the curriculum and the methodology for an educational approach to helping families with a mentally ill relative. The author explores an understanding of the current cultural context for providing services to the mentally ill, and understanding of the people being helped. These concepts are developed along with the related concepts of family consultation and psychoeducation. Provided is a knowledge base from which family educators can select curriculum content based on what families express as their needs. Also established are basic principles of adult learning and guidelines for effective and efficient learning.

*Hatfield, Agnes B. (1987). *Families of the mentally ill: Coping and adaptation.* New York: Guilford. (336 pgs).

>A number of aspects of coping and adaptation for families of the mentally ill are covered in this guide. It begins with a historical perspective of family caregivers, culture and mental illness, and a model of effective coping, and moves on to a discussion of how families cope with mental illness. Behavioral manifestations, family responses, social support, and coping strategies are explored. New perspectives on service provision and research are also mentioned.

Lafond, Virginia (1994). *Grieving mental illness: A guide for patients and their caregivers.* Canada: University of Toronto Press. (95 pgs).

>This is a self-help book for anyone who has experienced the effects of mental illness as a sufferer, family member, friend or caregiver. The author offers advice on how to move forward from a mental illness. She states, "By consciously grieving we can help bring healing and wholeness to our lives, resulting in new ways of coping, reduced stress, and greater self-esteem." Self-help exercises are included.

Ross, Jerilyn (1994). *Triumph over fear: A book of help and hope for people with anxiety, panic attacks, and phobias.* New York, NY: Bantam Books. (296 pgs).

>Jerilyn Ross overcame her own phobia to become one of the nation's leading authorities on anxiety disorders, panic attacks and phobias. In this comforting and inspiring book, she offers facts and techniques that can bring relief in a matter of weeks, no matter how long one has been suffering. Through fascinating case histories, she explores the many

faces of anxiety and introduces the step-by-step treatment plans that have worked for her patients.

*Todd, Tracy (1994). *Surviving & prospering in the managed mental health care marketplace.* Sarasota, FL: Professional Resource Press. (85 pgs).

This book was written to help mental health care providers understand the current situation regarding their profession, and to develop strategies for coping with legislative changes. Topics include: understanding managed care systems, identifying and applying to provider networks, getting referrals, making adjustments as a therapist, impacted disciplines, the role of employee assistance programs, and questions and answers. Appendices include a sample marketing letter, questions to ask the managed care system, a checklist for billing considerations, and sample managed care practice assessments.

Woolis, Rebecca (1992). *When someone you love has a mental illness: A handbook for family, friends, and caregivers.* New York, NY: Putnam Books. (232 pgs).

This guide addresses daily problems of living with a person with mental illness, as well as long-term planning and care. Of special note are the forty-three "Quick Reference Guides" dealing with such topics as: responding to hallucinations, delusions, violence and anger; helping your loved one comply with treatment and medication plans; deciding where the person should live; and choosing a doctor. The book is intended to be used as a handbook by families and friends of people with mental illness to help them understand that person and how to deal with him/her day-to-day.

Schizophrenia

*Anderson, Carol M., Reiss, Douglas J., & Hogarty, Gerard E. (1986). *Schizophrenia and the family: A practitioner's guide to psychoeducation and management.* New York, NY: Guilford Press. (365 pgs).

The authors approach schizophrenia from a psychoeducational approach taking into account the family's role as primary caretaker. The process of developing a productive treatment relationship with the patient and family is explored, and training issues and other applications of the psychoeducational model are addressed.

Backlar, Patricia (1994). *The family face of schizophrenia.* New York, NY: Jeremy P. Tarcher/Putnam. (283 pgs).

Patricia Backlar, a mental health ethicist and mother of a son who suffers from schizophrenia, eloquently recounts true stories about families whose adult children suffer from this cruel disease. Following each narrative, experts from various mental health professions offer advice on the issues raised by each story. This book teaches readers how to navigate the complicated labyrinth of medical and social services and to become more effective in managing schizophrenia.

Torrey, E. Fuller (1995). *Surviving schizophrenia: A manual for families, consumers and providers* (3rd ed.). New York, NY: HarperCollins Books. (409 pgs).

In clear language, this author describes the nature, causes, symptoms, treatment, and course of schizophrenia and also explores living with it from both the patient's and the family's point of view. This edition includes the latest research findings on what causes the disease as well as information about new drugs, and offers answers to frequently-asked questions.

Multiple Sclerosis

Carroll, David L. (1993). *Living well with MS.* New York: HarperCollins. (259 pgs)

Living Well with MS fills a strong need for a comprehensive book that will both comfort and inform the patient, family, and caregiver. The author carefully addresses topics such as diagnosis and prognosis, treatments for MS, exercises, diet, sexual dysfunction, emotional coping, and hope for a cure.

Kalb, Rosalind C., & Scheinberg, Labe C. (1992). *Multiple Sclerosis and the family.* New York: Demos Publications. (118 pgs)

This book includes discussions from experts in a variety of fields that explore the ways in which MS impacts the family group and describe strategies and resources that are available to more effectively help families manage their lives in the presence of MS. This volume will prove valuable to health care teams, professionals, and to individuals with MS and their families.

Parkinson's Disease

Atwood, Glenna W. (1991). *Living well with Parkinson's: An inspirational and informative guide for Parkinsonians and their loved ones.* New York, NY: John Wiley & Sons. (198 pgs).

> The author of this guide has Parkinson's Disease and has risen to national prominence as a leading spokesperson for Parkinson's. She tells of her personal struggles with this tragic disease and offers new hope to others who must face it. Atwood describes her intimate, proven prescriptions for living well with Parkinson's, including up-to-date information and guidance. For example, an appendix/directory lists the kinds of special clothing and equipment available and where to get them.

Hutton, Thomas J., & Pippel, Raye L. (1989). *Caring for the Parkinson patient.* Buffalo, NY: Prometheus Books. (196 pgs).

> This thoughtful collection of fourteen essays offers helpful information and useful suggestions relevant to virtually every concern voiced by parents, families, and caregivers. Experts in many fields contribute to provide information on topics such as new drug therapies, neural transplants, nursing techniques, exercises for movement and speech skills, how the disease impacts the family and where to seek help when support is needed.

Katz, Richard (1988). *Improving communication in Parkinson's disease.* Austin, TX: Pro-Ed. (25 pgs).

> The purpose of this booklet is to inform people about Parkinson's disease and to focus on one of its most common and painful problems, the breakdown in communication. It introduces and describes classic symptoms, speech characteristics, speech treatment, various types of difficulties and therapies, psychological considerations, and support groups and organizations.

Planning for the Future (Financial, Legal, Educational, etc.)

Berkobien, Richard (1991). *A family handbook on future planning.* Arlington, TX: Association for Retarded Citizens of the United States. (133 pgs).

> This manual is a comprehensive source of information on planning the future for a loved one, especially one with a physical or mental disability. It includes making financial arrangements; writing a will and/or letter of intent; answers questions about education, employment, financial support, residential programs for people with disabilities; and presents materials for planning for the future. Income, asset, trust and will forms; addresses of places to send for materials; and check lists are included.

Cane, Michael Allan (1995). *The five-minute lawyer's guide to estate planning.* New York, NY: Dell. (223 pgs).

> This practical handbook answers questions every person has about personal estate issues. Caregivers often experience an added pressure to carefully plan ahead for the care and well-being of their care receivers. Some of the topics covered in this book include: estate planning goals; wills, trusts, and life insurance; durable powers of attorney; joint tenancy with right of survivorship; gifts to and care of minor children; gift, estate, and inheritance taxes; and probate procedures.

Goldfluss, Howard E. (1994). *Living wills and wills.* New York, NY: Wings Books (244 pgs).

> *Living wills and wills* is written by Judge Goldfluss to help people make sure their wishes are followed when they can no longer state their own desires or after their deaths. Readers will find information on living wills, rights of a patient under the Patient Self Determination Act, wills and trusts, beneficiaries, probate, living trusts, and addresses and phone numbers of bar associations in each state. A sample will and forms for living wills, Health Care Proxy, and Durable Powers of Attorney are also included.

Russell, L. Mark, Grant, Arnold E., Joseph, Suzanne M., & Fee, Richard W. (1994). *Planning for the future: Providing a meaningful life for a child with a disability after your death.* Evanston, IL: American Publishing Company. (416 pgs).

Planning for the future is full of practical ideas and important information. It is an essential guide to parents of children who have disabilities. The authors explain how to prepare a life plan, a letter of intent, and a special needs trust, as well as how to maximize the child's government benefits, avoid probate, reduce estate taxes, and protect against the devastating costs of old age.

Stroke

Collins, Ellwyn K. (1992). *Unprepared! A husband's story of coping with his wife's stroke.* Minneapolis, MN: Deaconess Press. (195 pgs).

Unprepared! is especially helpful and meaningful for men who find themselves in caregiving roles. Collins relates his experiences of suddenly assuming housekeeping duties and caregiving responsibilities after his wife's stroke. Readers learn how he dealt with his emotions, with practical matters (he even includes recipes with added bits of humor), and with the health care system and providers.

Paullin, Ellen (1988). *Ted's stroke: The caregiver's story.* Cabin John, MD: Seven Locks Press. (175 pgs).

A personal account written by the wife of a man who suffered a stroke. The book vividly recounts time spent in intensive care, therapy, convalescence and day-to-day coping. One chapter is written by a physician who discusses what causes strokes, what happens physiologically when they occur, and prevention and reduction of one's risks of having a stroke.

Support/Self-Help Groups

Fradkin, Louise, Liberti, Mirca, & Madara, Edward (1993). *Guide to starting a self-help support group for caregivers of the aged.* Levittown, PA: Children of Aging Parents (C.A.P.S.) (62 pgs).

This book was written to serve as a guide for persons interested in starting caregiver self-help support groups in their communities. It includes information on factors to consider before you begin, how to start and keep a group going, and what to do at meetings. Appendices include information ranging from sample forms and discussion questions to information on resources. Also included are pages on a variety of elder care topics that can be copied and used as handouts for group members.

Hill, Karen (1987). *Helping you helps me: A guide book for self-help groups.* (2nd ed.). Ottawa, Ontario: Canadian Council on Social Development. (No page numbers).

This is a practical guide to starting and maintaining a self-help group. Leadership, membership, recruitment, fund-raising, problem-solving and decision-making are among the more than twenty topics covered.

*Katz, Alfred H., Hedrick, Hannah L., Isenberg, Daryl Holtz, Thompson, Leslie M., Goodrich, Therese, & Kutscher, Austin H. (Eds.). (1992). *Self-help: Concepts and applications.* Philadelphia, PA: Charles Press. (308 pgs).

The authors take a look at the severity of the need for self-help groups in America today. Self-help is discussed as it applies to specific diseases and medical conditions such as AIDS, Alzheimer's disease, multiple sclerosis, hearing loss, cancer, sudden infant death syndrome, etc. The authors explore the need for cooperation between organized medicine and self-help groups in the future of health care. Included is an analysis of how empowerment of individuals, families, and groups is fostered by self-help participation. This book will be an important resource both for self-help group activists and professional providers.

Powell, Thomas J. (Ed.). *Working with self-help.* Silver Spring, MD: National Association of Social Workers. (355 pgs).

This book is for persons interested in the self-help movement, either professionally or personally. Topics discussed include basic helping mechanisms common to different kinds of self-help programs, different types of self-help organizations, ways human service professionals can work with selected parts of the movement, clearinghouses, misuses of self-help, and use of self-help as an instrument for negotiating with professionals. Information is also provided on specific self-help groups and ways to enhance self-help activities in minority communities.

White, Barbara J., & Madara, Edward J. (Eds.). (1992). *The self-help sourcebook: Finding and forming mutual aid self-help groups* (4th ed.). Denville, NJ: Saint Clares-Riverside Medical Center. (208 pgs).

> This book is for individuals who are looking for a group to meet their special needs, professionals seeking an appropriate referral point for a client or information about a problem, academicians and researchers who want local or national self-help group contacts and information, policy makers at all levels of government, and media people seeking personal reactions to recent crises. It includes information about self-help clearinghouses, toll-free help lines, national self-help groups/organizations, resources for rare and genetic disorders, and information on the "how-tos" of starting and running local self-help groups.

*Wuthnow, Robert (1994). *Sharing the journey: Support groups and America's new quest for community*. Riverside, NJ: Free Press. (463 pgs).

> The author reports on a definitive and illuminating study of the phenomenon of support groups in America. Wuthnow examines the growth of the support group movement and its meaning in our national life. *Sharing the journey* illustrates how support groups develop, function, and serve the community. The possibilities and dangers of building community through support groups are explored. This book will provide new insights for anyone who wants to understand why small groups are a powerful source of identity in America today.

APPENDIX C
National Sources of Help for Caregivers

The Rosalynn Carter Institute has compiled this list of agencies, organizations, and services that can provide information to individuals who are caring for persons with physical or mental illnesses, difficulties of the frail elderly, or developmental disabilities. With the exception of "helplines" or "hotlines," each listing includes a complete mailing address and telephone numbers, and a brief description of the services or assistance provided.

The agencies and organizations included in the list are arranged alphabetically in three different sections. Section I, **GENERAL**, includes agencies/organizations which address a broad range of issues, disabilities, or illnesses. The second section, **AGING**, includes agencies and organizations that focus on aging, the elderly, and related issues. Section III, **SPECIFIC DISABILITIES AND DISEASES**, is arranged alphabetically by names of diseases, disabilities, or disorders. Please see the Table of Contents for specific diseases, illnesses, and disabilities included in Section III.

This information is provided in an effort to offer assistance to caregivers without the intention to endorse any particular agency or organization included on the list. Program leaders and participants may be aware of helpful resources which do not appear on this list. You are encouraged to ask the program leader or other representatives of organizations in your community about resources available for caregivers.

Contents

SECTION I
General   86

SECTION II
Aging   90

SECTION III
AIDS   92

Alcoholism/Substance Abuse   93

Allergies/Asthma   93

Alzheimer's Disease and Related Disorders   93

Amputation   93

Amyotrophic Lateral Sclerosis   93

Arthritis   93

Attention Deficit Disorder   94

Autism   94

Blindness   94

Cancer   94

Cerebral Palsy   95

Cystic Fibrosis   95

Deafness   95

Diabetes   96

Down Syndrome   96

Drug/Substance Abuse   96

Eating Disorders   96

Epilepsy   97

Head Injury   97

Heart Disorders   97

Hemophilia   97

Hydrocephalus   97

Incontinence   97

Kidney Disorders   97

Learning Disabilities   97

Leukemia   98

Lung Disease   98

Lupus   98

Mental Health   98

Mental Retardation   98

Multiple Sclerosis   98

Muscular Dystrophy	99	Spina Bifida	99
Neurological Disorders	99	Spinal Cord Injury	99
Parkinson's Disease	99	Stroke	99
Sickle Cell Disease	99	Visual Impairment	100

SECTION I

General

American Suicide Foundation
1045 Park Avenue
New York, NY 10028
(212) 410-1111; (800) 531-4477

Provides a way for business, community and professional leaders to find ways to fund suicide research, education, and prevention programs.

Administration for Children and Families
U.S. Dept. of Health and Human Services
370 L'Enfant Promenade, S.W.
Washington, DC 20447
(202) 401-9215

Oversees federal programs which promote the economic and social well-being of families and children.

Administration on Developmental Disabilities
U.S. Dept. of Health and Human Services
370 L'Enfant Promenade, S.W.
Washington, DC 20447
(202) 401-9215

Plans and carries out programs which promote the self-sufficiency and protect the rights of Americans with developmental disabilities.

American Association of Pastoral Counselors
9504-A Lee Highway
Fairfax, VA 22031
(703) 385-6967; (703) 352-7725 FAX

Provides clarity in pastoral counseling practice and training, criteria for religious institutions in pastoral counseling ministry, and coordination with other mental health professions.

ARCH National Resource Center
Chapel Hill Training-Outreach Project
800 Eastowne Drive, Suite 105
Chapel Hill, NC 27514-2215
(919) 490-5577; (800) 473-1727;
(919) 490-4905 FAX

Provides information, training, technical assistance, evaluation, and research activities to service providers, families and states in developing and maintaining respite services. Designed to create a nationwide service system of respite options.

Center for Family Support (mentally disabled)
386 Park Avenue, South
New York, NY 10016
(212) 889-5464; (212) 481-1082 FAX

Provides trained professionals to give caregivers respite; classes to teach parenting skills to persons with developmental disabilities; social activities for persons with developmental disabilities; and support groups for caregivers.

Children's Defense Fund
25 E Street, NW
Washington, DC 20001
(202) 628-8787; (202) 662-3510 FAX

Provides education about the needs of children and encourages preventative investment in children.

Children's Hospice International
901 N. Washington Street, Suite 700
Alexandria, VA 22314
(800) 242-4453; (703) 684-0330;
(703) 684-0226 FAX

Provides medical, psychological, emotional, and spiritual support to children with life-threatening conditions and their families.

Choice in Dying
200 Varick Street, Room 1001
New York, NY 10014
(212) 366-5540; (212) 765-8441 FAX

An educational and advocacy organization dedicated to the advancement of individual choice regarding end-of-life issues.

Clearinghouse on Disability Information
Office of Special Education & Rehabilitative Services
U.S. Department of Education
Room 3132, Switzer Building
Washington, DC 20202-2425
(202) 205-8241; (202) 205-8723 TTY

Responds to inquiries and provides referrals and information about services for individuals with disabilities at the national, state, and local level. Ask for "*The Pocket Guide to Federal Help for Individuals with Disabilities*"

Council for Exceptional Children
1920 Association Drive
Reston, VA 22091-1589
(703) 620-3660; (703) 264-9494 FAX

Provides professional development opportunities; advocates for underserved individuals with exceptionalities; sets professional standards; and helps professionals obtain conditions and resources necessary for effective practice.

The Family Caregiver Alliance
(*formerly* The Family Survival Project)
425 Bush Street, Suite 500
San Francisco, CA 94108
(800) 445-8106 In California;
(415) 434-3388 Outside California;
(415) 434-3508 FAX

Operates an information clearinghouse on brain impairments and caregiving; develops and disseminates publications; coordinates training and education programs; and conducts applied research.

Federation for Children with Special Needs
95 Berkeley Street, Suite 104
Boston, MA 02116
(800) 331-0688; (617) 482-2915

Provides a variety of information, education, training, and support opportunities regarding educational, health, advocacy, and policy-making issues for children and youth with special needs.

Foundation for Hospice and Homecare
228 Seventh Street, S.E.
Washington, DC 20003
(202) 547-7424; (202) 547-3540 FAX

Establishes standards of care, develops programs to prepare caregivers, educates the public, and conducts research on aging, health, and social policies.

HEATH Resource Center
One DuPont Circle, Suite 800
Washington, DC 20036-1193
(800) 544-3284; (202) 939-9320;
(202) 833-4760 FAX

Collects and disseminates information about education after high school for individuals with disabilities.

Institute on Community Integration (UAP)
University of Minnesota
109 Pattee Hall; 150 Pillsbury Drive, SE
Minneapolis, MN 55455
(612) 624-4512; (612) 624-9344 FAX

Is focused on improving the quality and community orientation of professional services and social supports available to individuals with disabilities and their families. Has three core activities—interdisciplinary training, services and technical assistance, and research and dissemination—across four program areas: Early Childhood and Early Intervention Services; School Age Services; Transition and Employment Services; and Adult and Community Services.

Learning Disabilities Association of America
4156 Library Road
Pittsburgh, PA 15234-1349

Offers information on a variety of topics for persons with learning disabilities, their families and professionals.

March of Dimes Birth Defects Foundation
1275 Mamoroneck Ave.
White Plains, NY 10605
(914) 428-7100

Provides information and funds programs related to congenital defects and genetic disorders.

National Alliance of Breast Cancer Organizations (NABCO)
9 East 37th Street, 10th Floor
New York, NY 10016
(212) 889-0606; (212) 689-1213 FAX

Includes a network of over 300 breast cancer organizations including comprehensive cancer centers, private and government agencies, and professional organizations. Provides information, assistance and referral to anyone with questions about breast cancer.

National Alliance for the Mentally Ill (NAMI)
2101 Wilson Blvd., Suite 302
Arlington, VA 22201
(800) 950-NAMI; (703) 524-7600

Provides support and guidance, education and advocacy for persons with severe and persistent mental illness.

National Arthritis, Muscoloskeletal and Skin Diseases Information Clearinghouse
P.O. Box AMS
9000 Rockville Place
Bethesda, MD 20892
(301) 495-4484; (301) 587-4352 FAX

Provides information exchange network among health professionals, organizations, and voluntary associations seeking to combat arthritic, muscoloskeletal, and skin diseases.

National Association for Home Care (NAHC)
228 Seventh Street, S.E.
Washington, DC 20003
(202) 547-7424; (202) 547-3540 FAX

A national non-profit organization representing providers of home care and hospice service throughout the U.S.

National Association of Medical Equipment Suppliers (NAMES)
625 Slaters Lane, Suite 200
Alexandria, VA 22314
(703) 836-6263; (703) 836-6730 FAX

Promotes access to quality home medical equipment services as an integral part of our health care system.

National Center for Youth with Disabilities
University of Minnesota
420 Delaware Street, SE, Box 721
Minneapolis, MN 55455-0392
(612) 626-2825; (800) 333-6293;
(612) 626-2134 FAX

Provides information and a resource center focusing on adolescents with chronic illnesses and disabilities and the issues that surround their transition to adult life.

National Clearinghouse on Postsecondary Education for Individuals with Disabilities
HEATH Resource Center
1 Dupont Circle, Suite 800
Washington, DC 20036-1193
(202) 939-9320; (800) 54H-EATH;
(202) 833-4760 FAX

Provides information on all aspects of education and training beyond high school for people with disabilities.

National Council on Patient Information & Education
666 11th Street, NW, Suite 810
Washington, DC 20001
(202) 347-6711; (202) 638-0773 FAX

Prepares patients to work with health care providers and to follow medication therapy safely and effectively.

National Easter Seal Society
70 East Lake Street
Chicago, IL 60601
(312) 726-6200; (312) 726-4258 (TDD);
(800) 221-6827

Provides information, support and direct services for persons with varied disabilities and their families.

National Family Caregivers Association
9621 E. Bexhill Drive
Kensington, MD 20895
(301) 942-6430; (301) 942-2302 FAX

The National Family Caregivers Association (NFCA) is a not-for-profit membership organization dedicated to making life better for America's family caregivers. The Association offers a newsletter, peer support, books and cards for caregivers.

National Federation of Interfaith Volunteer Caregivers, Inc.
368 Broadway, Suite 103
P.O. Box 1939
Kingston, NY 12401
(914) 331-1358; (800) 350-7438
e-mail: nficvc@aol.com
www.nifvc.org

Assists congregations of all faiths to undertake ministry of caregiving to the frail elderly, disabled persons, and their families.

The National Home Caring Council
67 Irving Place
New York, NY 10003
(212) 674-4990

Provides information on appropriate in-home services.

National Hospice Organization (NHO)
1901 N. Moore Street, Suite 901
Arlington, VA 22209
(800) 658-8898 Helpline

Promotes quality care for terminally ill patients and provides information about hospice services available in the United States.

National Information Center for Children and Youth With Disabilities
P.O. Box 1492
Washington, DC 20013
(202) 884-8200; (202) 884-8441 (FAX);
(800) 695-0285

Provides free information on disabilities and disability-related issues.

National Information Clearinghouse for Infants with Developmental Disabilities and Life-Threatening Conditions
University of South Carolina
School of Medicine, Dept. of Pediatrics
Columbia, SC 29208
(800) 922-9234, ext. 201 (Voice & TT)

Provides assistance to meet the information needs of caregivers and to protect the rights of infants with disabilities and life-threatening conditions.

National Institute of Child Health and Human Development
(301) 496-3454

Provides information on current research and assistance regarding children's health and human development.

National Institute of Mental Health
U.S. Department of Health & Human Services
5600 Fishers Lane, Room 15C-05
Rockville, MD 20857
(800) 421-4211

Conducts and supports research to learn more about causes, prevention, and treatment of mental and emotional illnesses. Collects and distributes information related to mental illness. Free publications available on request.

National Institute on Community-Based Long-Term Care
c/o National Council on Aging (NCOA)
409 Third Street, SW
Washington, DC 20024
(202) 479-1200

Promotes consumer directed and consumer choice opportunities for adults with disabilities through education, training, and research.

National Insurance Consumer Helpline
(800) 942-4242

Provides printed information and answers questions regarding health, life, auto and home owners' insurance.

National Mental Health Consumer's Self-Help Clearinghouse
311 S. Juniper Street, Suite 1000
Philadelphia, PA 19107
(215) 735-6082; (215) 735-0275 FAX;
(800) 553-4539

Promotes and assists the development of consumer run self-help mental health groups.

The National Organization for Rare Disorders
P.O. Box 8923; 100 Route 37
New Fairfield, CT 06812-1783
(203) 746-6518; (800) 999-NORD

Is dedicated to finding effective treatment for patients with rare illnesses.

Older Women's League (O-W-L)
666 11th Street, NW, Suite 700
Washington, DC 20001
(202) 783-6686; (800) 825-3695;
(202) 638-2356 FAX

Advocates for women caregivers in their later years.

Parent Care
9041 Colgate Street
Indianapolis, IN 46268
(317) 872-9913 Phone & FAX

Provides information and support to families of infants who require special care at birth due to handicaps resulting from premature birth.

Parents Helping Parents
535 Race Street, Suite 120
San Jose, CA 95126
(408) 288-5010

Helps children with special needs receive care, services, and education. Provides education, support, and training for parents.

Rosalynn Carter Institute of Georgia Southwestern State University
600 Simmons Street
Americus, GA 31709
(912) 928-1234; (912) 931-2663 FAX

Provides information, educational programs, research and general assistance to family (informal) and professional (formal) caregivers of persons with mental and emotional problems, difficulties of the frail elderly, developmental disabilities, or physical illnesses.

Social Security Administration Hotline
(800) 772-1213; (800) 325-0778 (TTD)

Provide information and assist with questions about retirement, Supplemental Security Income (SSI), change of address and other concerns related to the Social Security Administration.

The Association for Persons with Severe Handicaps (TASH)
11201 Greenwood Avenue, North
Seattle, WA 98133
(206) 361-8870; (206) 361-9208 FAX

Provides information and support for parents of children with severe handicaps and profound retardation. Supports full inclusion for everyone in schools, the workplace, and the community, and advocates support to families and the closure of institutions.

The Well Spouse Foundation
P.O. Box 28876
San Diego, CA 92198
(619) 673-9043

Provides support and information for the well spouse of a chronically ill person. (The founder, Maggie Strong, is the author of the book *Mainstay*.)

SECTION II

Aging

Administration on Aging
330 Independence Avenue, SW, Suite 4760
Washington, DC 20201
(202) 619-0556

Develops federal government programs and coordinates community services for older people.

American Association of Homes and Services for the Aging (AAHSA)
901 E Street, NW, Suite 500
Washington, DC 20004
(202) 783-2242; (202) 783-2255 FAX

Includes not-for-profit organizations dedicated to providing high-quality health care, housing and community service primarily to the elderly. Offers a variety of for-sale publications, primarily for professionals.

American Association of Retired Persons (AARP)
601 E Street, NW
Washington, DC 20049
(800) 424-2277

Offers many free informational pamphlets such as "*The Caregiver Resource Kit*" (D15267), "*A Handbook About Care in the Home: Information on Home Care Services*", "*Nursing Home Life: A Guide for Residents and Families*", "*Medicare: What it Covers, What it Doesn't*", "*Miles Away and Still Caring: A Handbook for Long-Distance Caregivers*."

American Society on Aging
833 Market Street, Suite 511
San Francisco, CA 94130
(415) 974-9600

Provides the public with information about issues that affect older persons and promotes ways of meeting their needs.

Children of Aging Parents (C.O.A.P.)
1609 Woodbourne Road, Suite 302A
Levittown, PA 19057
(215) 945-6900

Helps caregivers cope with the stress of caregiving and provides support to them.

Commission on Legal Problems of the Elderly
1800 M Street, NW
Washington, DC 20036
(202) 331-2297

Analyzes and responds to the legal needs of older people in the United States.

Eldercare America
1141 Loxford Terrace
Silver Spring, MD 20901
(301) 593-1621

Advocates for long-term care and on behalf of caregivers; preserves the dignity and abilities of older persons.

Eldercare Locator
(800) 677-1116

Provides referrals to local community agencies for homecare and respite in conjunction with the U.S. Administration on Aging. Have available the address, including zip code, of older adult needing assistance when you call.

Mental Disorders of the Aging Research Branch
Division of Clinical Treatment Research
National Institute of Mental Health
5600 Fishers Lane, Room 18-105
Rockville, MD 20857
(301) 443-1185; (301) 594-6784 FAX

Supports a broad program of basic, clinical, and applied research, research training, and career development focusing on the nature, treatment, and prevention of major mental disorders and behavioral dysfunctions in later life.

National Alliance for Caregiving
4720 Montgomery Lane
Suite 642
Bethesda, MD 20814
(301) 718-8444
(301) 652-7711 FAX

The National Alliance for Caregiving (NAC) is a nonprofit partnership, created in 1996 to support family caregivers of the elderly and the professionals who serve them. The Alliance conducts research, develops national projects and works to increase public awareness of the issues of family caregiving.

National Association of Area Agencies on Aging
(NAAAA)
1112 16th Street, NW, Suite 100
Washington, DC 20036
(202) 296-8130; (202) 296-8134 FAX

Represents the interests of Area Agencies on Aging across the country. Guide to community resources.

National Council on the Aging, Inc. (NCOA)
409 3rd Street, SW, 2nd Floor
Washington, DC 20024
(202) 479-1200; (202) 479-6674 TDD;
(202) 479-0735 FAX

Serves as a national resource for information, technical assistance, training, and research related to the field of aging.

National Association of Professional Geriatric Care Managers
1604 North Country Club Road
Tucson, AZ 85716
(602) 881-8008

Assists older people and their families with long-term care arrangements.

National Eldercare Institute on Health Promotion and Aging
American Association of Retired Persons
601 E Street, NW, 5th Floor, Building B
Washington, DC 20049
(202) 434-2240; (202) 434-6474 FAX

Encourages healthy behaviors to reduce risk of chronic and preventable conditions, and to maintain and improve function among physically and/or mentally impaired older persons.

National Gerontological Nursing Association
7250 Parkway Drive, Suite 510
Hanover, MD 21076
(800) 723-0560

Develops and supports educational programs for nurses, health providers, and general public; provides a forum for the exchange of ideas; disseminates information and research on gerontological nursing to all interested persons.

National Institute of Mental Health Aging Branch
5600 Fishers Lane, Room 18-105
Rockville, MD 20857
(301) 443-1185

Conducts and supports research to learn more about the causes, prevention, and treatment of mental and emotional illnesses.

National Institute on Aging (NIA)
P.O. Box 8057
Gaithersburg, MD 20898-8057
(800) 222-2225; (800) 222-4225 (TDD)

Conducts and supports research and training related to aging processes and the diseases of older people. Provides publications on a variety of topics.

Senior Care Centers of America
26 E 2nd Street
Moorestown, NJ 08057
(609) 778-0624

Has Adult Day Health Care Centers with locations in several states, providing full supervisory services in a comfortable homelike atmosphere. Provides counseling, guidance, and information to assist the caregivers.

Shepherd's Centers of America
6700 Troost Ave., Suite 616
Kansas City, MO 64131

Assists and serves older adults in a variety of ways while also establishing and developing intentional ministries with older adults within a congregation. Individual centers intiate or terminate programs and services in response to identified needs and interests of people in their areas.

SECTION III
Specific Disabilities and Diseases
(Alphabetical by name of disorder)

AIDS

HIV Information Exchange and Support Group
610 Greenwood
Glenview, IL 60025
(708) 724-3832

Offers support groups and peer counseling based on adaptation of 12-step program.

Families Who Care
6475 Pacific Coast Hwy., Suite 202
Long Beach, CA 90803-4296
(310) 498-6366

Provides information on how to start your own AIDS family support group.

Mothers of AIDS Patients
1811 Field Drive, NE
Albuquerque, NM 87112
(619) 544-0430

Provides support for families of AIDS patients.

Pediatric AIDS Foundation
1311 Colorado Ave.
Santa Monica, CA 90404
(310) 395-9051; (310) 395-5149 FAX

Provides informational resources, free parent-education programs, emergency assistance grants, research into blocking transmission from pregnant mothers to newborns, and research grants and scholar awards.

The CDC National AIDS Hotline
P.O. Box 6003
Rockville, MD 20850
(800) 342-AIDS;
(800) 344-7432 (Hispanic);
(800) 243-7889 (Hearing Impaired)

Provides HIV/AIDS information, education, and referral service for the United States.

Alcoholism/Substance Abuse

National Council on Alcoholism and Drug Dependence, Inc.
12 West 21 Street
New York, NY 10010
(212) 206-6770; (212) 645-1690 (FAX);
(800) NCA-CALL

Seeks to prevent disease of alcoholism, other drug addictions and related problems through public education and research; advocates on behalf of alcoholics and their families; provides publications and referrals to local affiliates.

Allergies/Asthma

American Allergy Association
P.O. Box 7273
Menlo Park, CA 94026-7273
or
1259 El Camino #254
Menlo Park, CA 94025

Offers publications and resource material related to allergies and asthma. Services include information on living with allergies, data searches, allergy information sheets, and medication and tests for asthma.

Alzheimer's Disease and Related Disorders

Alzheimer's Disease and Related Disorders Association, Inc.
919 N. Michigan Ave., Suite 1000
Chicago, IL 60611-1676
(312) 335-8700; (800) 272-3900

Carries out its mission in five primary areas: research, education of the public, chapter formation for a nationwide family support network, advocacy for improved public policy and legislation, and patient and family services. Sponsors public education programs and offers supportive services to patients and families coping with Alzheimer's disease.

Alzheimer's Disease Education & Referral Center
P.O. Box 8250
Silver Spring, MD 20907-8250
(800) 438-4380; (301) 587-4352 FAX
Collects, stores, and distributes information concerning Alzheimer's disease for health professionals, patients and their families, and the general public.

Amputation

National Amputation Foundation
73 Church Street
Malverne, NY 11565
(516) 887-3600; (516) 887-3667
Provides legal counsel, vocational guidance and placement, psychological aid, and training in the use of prosthetic devices.

Amyotrophic Lateral Sclerosis (A.L.S.) *(Lou Gehrig's Disease)*

A.L.S. and Neuromuscular Research Foundation
3698 California Street, Room 548
San Francisco, CA 94118
(415) 923-3640
Provides diagnostic & treatment services for with ALS; conducts clinical trials of experimental therapies; offers support group meetings, video lending library, and equipment loan program.

A.L.S. Association
21021 Ventura Blvd.
Woodland Hills, CA 91364
(818) 340-7500
Provides information, a referral service, support groups, and counseling.

Arthritis

Arthritis Foundation
2045 Peachtree Road, Suite 800
Atlanta, GA 30309
(404) 872-7100

Provides information and support to persons with rheumatic diseases and their families.

Attention Deficit Disorder

National Attention Deficit Disorder Association (NADDA)
(for information on local support groups)
19262 Jamboree Road
Irvine, CA 92715
(for membership in NADDA)
P.O. Box 488
West Newbury, MA 01985
(800) 487-2282

Provides services including referrals to local support groups, distribution of resource materials, and conferences.

Autism

Autism Network International
P.O. Box 1545
Lawrence, KS 66044

Offers support and information on referrals, problem solving, treatments and therapies, and services for persons with autism.

Autism Society of America
7910 Woodmont Avenue, Suite 650
Bethesda, MD 20814
(800) 3AU-TISM (328-8476);
(301) 657-0881; (301) 657-0869 FAX

Provides facts on all aspects of autism to parents, professionals, and public.

National Autism Hotline
(304) 525-8014

Provides information, referrals, advocacy and other services related to the needs of people with autism and similar disabilities.

Blindness

American Council of the Blind
1155 15th Street, NW, Suite 720
Washington, DC 20005
(202) 467-5081; (800) 424-8666

Provides information and advocacy for individuals who are blind, visually impaired, or deaf-blind, and their families.

American Foundation for the Blind
15 W. 16th Street
New York, NY 10011
(800) AF-BLIND; (212) 620-2000

Provides "The Directory of Services for the Visually Impaired," a state-by-state listing of services available nationally.

Cancer

American Cancer Society
1599 Clifton Road, NE
Atlanta, GA 30329
(800) 227-2345

Provides support and direct services to persons with cancer and their families.

Breast Cancer Advisory Center
P.O. Box 224
Kensington, MD 20895
(301) 949-2531; (301) 949-1132 FAX

Publishes brochure, "If you've thought about breast cancer."

Cancer Care
(212) 221-3300

Provides counseling, information, referral and educational programs regarding cancer care.

Cancer Information Services
Office of Cancer Communications
National Cancer Institute/National Institutes of Health
Building 31, 10A24
9000 Rockville Pike
Bethesda, MD 20892
(800) 422-6237

Answers questions and offers publications about various aspects of cancer: prevention, detection, causes, and treatment.

Candlelighters Childhood Cancer Foundation
7910 Woodmont Ave., Suite 460
Bethesda, MD 20892
(301) 657-8401; (800) 366-2223 CCCF;
(301) 718-2686 FAX

Provides learning and support for families with children or adolescents with cancer.

Chemocare (Cancer)
(800) 55-CHEMO;
(908) 233-1103 in New Jersey

Matches cancer patients with volunteers who have had a similar diagnosis. Volunteers provide emotional support on the phone or in person, if possible. A national agency.

National Alliance of Breast Cancer Organizations (NABCO)
1180 Avenue of the Americas, 2nd Floor
New York, NY 10036
(212) 719-0154

Provides a clearinghouse for breast cancer information.

National Cancer Institute
(800) 4-CANCER

Provides cancer information.

National Children's Cancer Society
1015 Locust Street, Suite 1040
St. Louis, MO 63101-1323
(800) 532-6459; (314) 241-1600

Provides financial assistance for bone marrow transplant, donor harvest, donor search, donor recruitment, tissue typing.

The Wellness Community, National
2716 Ocean Park Blvd., Suite 1030
Santa Monica, CA 90405
(310) 314-2555; (310) 314-7586 FAX

Provides psychosocial support groups for cancer patients and their families in a limited number of cities.

Cerebral Palsy

United Cerebral Palsy Association
1522 K Street, NW, #1112
Washington, DC 20005
(800) 872-5827; (202) 842-1266;
(202) 842-3519 FAX

Provides information, support, and direct services to persons with cerebral palsy and other neuromotor disabilities and their families.

Cystic Fibrosis

Cystic Fibrosis Foundation
6931 Arlington Road
Bethesda, MD 20814
(800) FIGHT-CF;
(301) 951-4422; (301) 951-6378 FAX

Provides information and support for families of children with this chronic degenerative disease.

Deafness

American Society for Deaf Children (ASDC)
2848 Arden Way, Suite 210
Sacramento, CA 95825-1373

Provides information and support to parents of children who are deaf or hearing impaired; referral to local resources; linkage with deaf adults; newsletters.

National Association of the Deaf (NAD)
814 Thayer Avenue
Silver Spring, MD 20910-4500
(301) 587-1788; (301) 587-1789 (TDD);
(301) 587-1791 FAX

Provides information, support and advocacy for persons who are deaf or hearing impaired.

National Information Center on Deafness
Gallaudet University
800 Florida Ave., NE
Washington, DC 20002
(202) 651-5051; (202) 651-5052 TTY;
(202) 651-5054 FAX

Provides objective information dealing with deafness and hearing loss, including devices, communication strategies, coping strategies.

Self Help for Hard of Hearing People, Inc. (SHHH)
7910 Woodmont Ave., Suite 1200
Bethesda, MD 20814
(301) 657-2248; (301) 657-2249 (TDD);
(301) 913-9413 FAX

Provides information and support to persons with hearing impairment and their families.

Diabetes

American Diabetes Association
National Service Center
1660 Duke Street
Alexandria, VA 22314
(800) 232-3472; (703) 549-1500;
(703) 683-2890 FAX

Provides information and support to persons with diabetes and their families.

Juvenile Diabetes Foundation International
432 Park Avenue, South, 16th Floor
New York, NY 10016
(800) 533-2873 (JDF-CURE);
(212) 889-7575; (212) 532-8791 FAX

Provides information and support to families of children with juvenile diabetes.

National Diabetes Information Clearinghouse
Box NDIC
9000 Rockville Pike
Bethesda, MD 20892
(301) 654-3327

Offers information about diabetes to health professionals, patients, and the general public.

Down Syndrome

Association for Children with Down Syndrome
2616 Martin Ave.
Bellmore, NY 11710
(516) 221-4700; (516) 221-4311 FAX

Provides families with individual and group support, home and hospital visitations, and special events throughout the school year.

National Down Syndrome Society
666 Broadway
New York, NY 10012
(800) 221-4602; (212) 460-9330;
(212) 979-2873 FAX

Provides information and support for families of children with Down Syndrome. Supports research, provides services for families and individuals.

Parents of Down Syndrome Children
11600 Nebel Street
Rockville, MD 20852
(301) 984-5792

Provide advocacy and direct services to people with Down Syndrome and their families.

Drug/Substance Abuse

National Council on Alcoholism and Other Drug Dependencies
12 West 21st Street
New York, NY 10010
(212) 206-6770

Educates the public about the disease of alcoholism and other drug dependencies. Promotes programs for prevention.

Eating Disorders

National Association of Anorexia Nervosa and Associated Disorders (ANAD)
Box 7
Highland Park, IL 60035
(708) 831-3438; (708) 433-4632

Provides a number of programs and services for persons with eating disorders (anorexia, bulimia, binge eating) and their families. These programs/services include counseling, self-help groups, educational programs and referrals.

Epilepsy

Epilepsy Foundation of America
4351 Garden City Drive
Landover, MD 20785
(800) EFA-1000; (301) 459-3700;
(301) 577-2684 FAX

Provides information and support to persons with epilepsy and seizure disorders and their families.

Head Injury

National Head Injury Foundation
1776 Massachusetts Ave, NW, Suite 100
Washington, DC 20036
(202) 296-6443; (800) 444-6443;
(202) 296-8850 FAX

Provides information and support to persons with head injuries and their families.

Heart Disorders

American Heart Association
7272 Greenville Ave.
Dallas, TX 75231-4596
(214) 373-6300; (214) 706-1341 FAX

Provides information to persons with cardiovascular disorders, stroke, or aphasia.

Hemophilia

National Hemophilia Foundation (NHF)
110 Greene Street, Room 303
New York, NY 10012
(212) 431-8541; (212) 431-0906 FAX;
(800) 42-HANDI

Provides information and support to persons with hemophilia (and other clotting factor deficiencies) and their families.

Hydrocephalus

National Hydrocephalus Foundation
400 N. Michigan Ave., Suite 1102
Chicago, IL 60611-4102
(815) 467-6548

Provides information for families of children with hydrocephalus.

Incontinence

Help for Incontinent People
P.O. Box 544
Union, SC 29379
(803) 579-7900; (800) BLADDER (252-3337);
(803) 579-7902 FAX

Provides education, advocacy and support to the public and health professionals about the prevalence, causes, prevention, diagnosis, treatment and management alternatives for incontinence.

Kidney Disorders

National Kidney Foundation
30 East 33rd Street, 11th Floor
New York, NY 10016
(800) 622-9010; (212) 889-2210

Provides information and support to persons with diseases of the kidney and urinary tract, and their families.

Learning Disabilities

Learning Disabilities Association of America
4156 Library Road
Pittsburgh, PA 15234
(412) 341-1515; (412) 341-8077;
(412) 344-0224 FAX

Provides information and support to persons with learning disabilities and their families.

Leukemia

Children's Leukemia Research Association
585 Stewart Avenue, Suite 536
Garden City, NY 11530
(516) 222-1944

Raises funds to support research efforts into the causes and cure of leukemia and to provide patient aid to those families in need while meeting the expenses incurred in leukemia treatment.

Leukemia Society of America
600 3rd Ave.
New York, NY 10016
(212) 573-8484; (800) 955-4LSA

Provides information and support to persons with leukemia, the lymphomas, multiple myeloma, and Hodgkin's Disease. Local chapters have patient aid programs that provide funds for treatment and other services.

National Leukemia Association
585 Stewart Avenue, Suite 536
Garden City, NY 11530
(516) 222-1944

Provides patient aides, assistance with medications, diagnostic tests, and lab fees for persons with leukemia.

Lung Disease

American Lung Association
1740 Broadway
New York, NY 10019
(212) 315-8700; (212) 265-5642 FAX

Provides information on respiratory conditions such as tuberculosis, bronchitis, asthma, and emphysema.

Lupus

Lupus Foundation of America, Inc.
Columbus Chapter
P.O. Box 12412
Columbus, GA 31907-1012
(706) 571-8950

Provides current literature about Lupus; conducts monthly support group meetings; publishes a quarterly newsletter; and raises funds for awareness, education and research.

Mental Health

National Mental Health Association
1021 Prince Street
Alexandria, VA 22314-2971
(703) 838-7521; (703) 684-5968 FAX

Provides information on numerous problems and issues related to mental health in children and adults. Brochures available on such topics as depression, suicide, schizophrenia, and stress.

Mental Retardation

American Association on Mental Retardation
1719 Kalorama Road, NW
Washington, DC 20009
(202) 387-1968

Enhances life opportunities for people with mental retardation by exchanging information that advances the skills and knowledge of individuals in the field.

The ARC National Headquarters
500 E. Border Street, Suite 300
Arlington, TX 76010
or
P.O. Box 1047
Arlington, TX 76004
(817) 261-6003; (817) 277-0553 (TDD)

Provides information and support to persons with mental retardation and their families; seeks to ensure the rights of people with mental retardation.

Multiple Sclerosis

Multiple Sclerosis Foundation
6350 N. Andrews Ave.
Fort Lauderdale, FL 33309
(305) 776-6805; (800) 441-7055;
(305) 938-8708 FAX

Provides information on legal rights, diet and nutrition; general infomation about coping with MS; and traditional and alternative health care treatments.

National Multiple Sclerosis Society
733 3rd Ave.
New York, NY 10017
(212) 986-3240; (800) FIGHT-MS;
(212) 986-7981 FAX

Provides information, support, and direct services for persons with multiple sclerosis, related diseases, and their families.

Muscular Dystrophy

Muscular Dystrophy Association
3300 E. Sunrise Drive
Tucson, AZ 85718
(602) 529-2000

Maintains a worldwide research effort, a nationwide program of medical services, and professional and public health education.

Neurological Disorders

National Institute of Neurological Disorders and Stroke
9000 Rockville Pike, Bldg 31, Room 8A-16
Bethesda, MD 20892
(301) 496-5751; (800) 352-9424;
(301) 402-2186 FAX

Is the principal agency for research on the causes, prevention, detection, and treatment of neurological diseases and stroke.

Parkinson's Disease

National Parkinson's Foundation
1501 NW Ninth Ave.
Miami, FL 33136
(800) 327-4545; (800) 433-7022 in FL;
(800) 400-8448 in CA

Works to find cause and cure of Parkinson's Disease, educates patients and public, and provides diagnostic & therapeutic services.

Sickle Cell Disease

Sickle Cell Disease Association of America
200 Corporate Pointe, Suite 49
Culver City, CA 90230-7633
(800) 421-8453

Distributes educational materials; trains sickle cell trait counselors; conducts patient, professional and public education programs; provides technical assistance for programs designed to meet the needs of persons with sickle cell conditions.

Spina Bifida

Spina Bifida Association of America
4590 MacArthur Blvd., NW #250
Washington, DC 20007-4226
(800) 621-3141; (202) 944-3285;
(202) 944-3295 FAX

Provides information and support to families of children with spina bifida and related hydrocephalus.

Spinal Cord Injury

National Spinal Cord Injury Hotline
Monkbello Hospital
2201 Argonne Drive
Baltimore, MD 21218
(800) 526-3456

Provides toll-free information and referral service. Available to individuals who have sustained a traumatic spinal cord injury and their families. Office hours are Monday–Friday, 9:00 a.m.–5:00 p.m. EST (24 hours for new injuries).

Stroke

Courage Stroke Network
3915 Golden Valley Road
Golden Valley, MN 55422
(612) 520-0524; (800) 553-6321;
(612) 520-0577 FAX

Provides a communication link for stroke survivors, their family members, and professionals to share information on stroke and experiences related to stroke.

National Stroke Association
8480 E. Orchard Road, Suite 1000
Englewood, CO 80111-5015
(303) 771-1700; (800) STR-OKES;
(303) 771-1887 TDD; (303) 771-1886 FAX

Provides information about stroke to the general public and professionals and offers supportive services to stroke survivors and their families.

Stroke Connection
American Heart Association
7272 Greenville Avenue
Dallas, TX 75231-4596

Is a nationwide resource for stroke survivors, their families and professionals. Provides toll-free stroke information and referral line, referral to local stroke support groups, assistance in developing stroke groups, and education and information.

Visual Impairment

Lighthouse National Center for Vision and Aging
800 Second Avenue
New York, NY 10017
(212) 808-0077; (800) 334-5497;
(212) 808-0110 FAX; (212) 808-5544 TTY-TTD

Promotes interest of older people with, or at risk of incurring, vision impairment.

National Association for Parents of the Visually Impaired (NAPVI)
P.O. Box 317
Watertown, MA 02272-0317
(800) 562-6265

Provides support for parents of children who have visual impairments or multiple disabilities.

National Association for Visually Handicapped (NAVH)
22 West 21st Street, 6th Floor
New York, NY 10010
(212) 889-3141; (202) 727-2931 FAX

Provides information, referral, and direct services for persons with partial vision and their families.

The Authors

~

David H. Haigler, Ed.D., is Deputy Director of the Rosalynn Carter Institute of Georgia Southwestern State University. He is a Licensed Master Social Worker (LMSW) in Georgia with over twenty years of experience in mental health and human services. Dr. Haigler is co-author of *Characteristics, Concerns, and Concrete Needs of Formal and Informal Caregivers: Understanding and Appreciating Their Marathon Existence*, issued by Georgia Southwestern State University; and he is a contributing author of *Caring and Competent Caregivers*, published by the University of Georgia Press. He received his Ed.D. in curriculum and supervision from the University of Georgia.

Kathryn Beckham Mims, Ph.D., is Director of Senior Adult Ministries at First Baptist Church in Albany, Georgia, and guest faculty member for Family Information Services of Minneapolis, Minnesota. Her previous positions include Professional Associate at the Rosalynn Carter Institute, and Assistant Professor and Extension Family Life Specialist at both Kansas State University and the Ohio State University. She served as the state coordinator of the Volunteer Information Provider Project (VIPP), an information program for caregivers of elderly adults, while in Kansas and for the Senior Series Project in Ohio. She received her Ph.D. in child and family development and a Certificate in Gerontology from the University of Georgia and is a Licensed Master Social Worker (LMSW) in the State of Georgia.

Jack A. Nottingham, Ph.D., is Executive Director of the Rosalynn Carter Institute of Georgia Southwestern State University. He has held professorships in psychology at the University of Maryland International Division, Western Michigan University, and the University of Hawaii. He is co-editor of *The Professional and Family Caregiver—Dilemmas, Rewards and New Directions*, issued by Georgia Southwestern State University; and co-author of *Caring and Competent Caregivers* published by the University of Georgia Press. Dr. Nottingham is a licensed psychologist in the State of Georgia. He received his Ph.D. in psychology from George Peabody College of Vanderbilt University.